ANXIOUS to UNSHAKEABLE

DISCOVER YOUR ANXIETY TYPE, CONQUER YOUR STRESS, AND GAIN *Peace of Mind*

David Olson

Copyright © 2025 by David Olson

All rights reserved.

No portion of this book may be reproduced in any form without written permission from the publisher or author, except as permitted by U.S. copyright law.

This publication is designed to provide accurate and authoritative information in regard to the subject matter covered. It is sold with the understanding that neither the author nor the publisher is engaged in rendering specific, individualized medical advice. While the publisher and author have used their best efforts in preparing this book, they make no representations or warranties with respect to the accuracy or completeness of the contents of this book and specifically disclaim any implied warranties of merchantability or fitness for a particular purpose.

Book Cover by LSDesign, 99designs.

Contents

Acknowledgements	1
Introduction	2
1. The Function of Anxiety and How It Can Go Wrong	4
2. A Toolbox for Defeating Dysfunctional Anxiety	11
3. The Anxieties of Modern Living	34
4. Type 1: Generalized Anxiety	51
5. Type 2: Phobias	62
6. Type 3: Post Traumatic Stress	74
7. Type 4: Social Anxiety	86
8. Type 5: Panic Attacks	97
9. Type 6: Anxious Attachment Style	108
10. Type 7: Existential Anxiety	127
11. Substance Abuse and Its Relationship With Anxiety	140
12. Sticking Points, Final Thoughts	154
13. References	167

Acknowledgements

When I sat down to write this book, I came with the intention of making it one of my life's great achievements, and if it indeed reaches the success that I hope it will be and touches the lives of many people in the world, I wouldn't want to have passed up on the opportunity to acknowledge the many individuals who have made this book possible. My most sincere wish for everyone in the world is that they will have the kind of people in their lives to love, support, and inspire them the way that I have been by the people close to me. With that said, I want to thank and acknowledge some very special individuals in my life.

I want to acknowledge the love and support of my parents, Richard and Carol. I owe everything that I have to them and they are role models in the truest sense of the word. I want to acknowledge my brothers, as well, for their constant support, encouragement, and feedback throughout my life. A man could not ask for better siblings.

I want to acknowledge my teachers and professors, for all the time and effort that they invested in me over the years. I want to thank them for believing in me and challenging me to be a better student and person.

I want to acknowledge my mentors. These are the people that took me in, taught me everything that they knew, respected me, and believed in me during the process. These people are: Amy, from the world of track and field; Vanessa, when I was working in the school system; and Felica, from my time working in the clinical setting. You all taught me so much.

Lastly, I wanted to thank my assistant, Maya. Our numerous brainstorming sessions were instrumental in shaping and developing this book into what it is now.

Introduction

If you have picked up this book out of curiosity, wondering what it's all about and how it can benefit you, I thought I'd do you a favor and include an introduction section which answers that question. My name is David Olson, and I've been around the world of psychology since I was but a sophomore in college, which is to say for about a quarter of a century now. I've worked in the hospital setting, administering psychological tests. I've taught college courses on psychology. I've worked in the school setting doing behavioral intervention, and I have worked as a counselor in the clinical setting. I was driven to write this book, because the majority of the clients that I have worked with professionally were dealing with severe anxiety issues and I have come to realize just how common of a problem it is in the general public. I have even had to deal with my own anxiety flare-ups and have family members that sometimes struggle to manage the severity of anxiety that they often experience. What I want to give the world is a book that helps people think about their relationship to anxiety, how to identify the types of anxiety that they may experience, and how to use the best tools available in the field to resolve their anxiety in a functional manner.

In the early chapters of this book, we will address the issue of anxiety on a philosophical level, investigating a variety of questions: What is anxiety? Why do we experience it? What purpose does it serve? How do we develop a good relationship with our anxiety? We will also address a lot of the ways that our environment evokes feelings of anxiety. From there, we will be exploring what to do about our anxiety, and learn some of the different tools that psychologists and their patients have used to address severe anxiety. After we have dipped our toes into the subject of anxiety resolution, we will begin to address some of the more specific forms of anxiety. These are diagnosable disorders of anxiety, found in the APA's Diagnostic and Statistical Manual of Mental Disorders, 5th edition. We will address the symptoms of these specific anxiety disorders and at the end of each of these chapters, I will make recommendations for which tools will likely be the most effective in addressing and resolving that specific type of anxiety disorder.

Stylistically, I have attempted to write a book that is accessible to just about anyone. I have endeavored to stay away from using fancy psychology lingo, buzzwords, and generally pretentious language. I want this to be a book that people who come from all walks of life can read, enjoy, and learn from. Throughout this book, I have also included a number of references to events in my own life, or references to work I have done with past clients. This is to help the book feel more authentic and practical. Any events that I make reference to are all real events, but in the case of my clients, I have excluded any identifying information that would jeopardize confidentiality.

I have also included some bonus features with this book, which I am excited about. Along with the book, I have constructed a Facebook group and YouTube channel, which are associated with the book. This is so that you can get additional information, resources, and connect with other individuals, including myself. I will be including a password code to get into the Facebook group. You will see it in a later chapter.

Finally, I want to give advice as to how to read this book. Some people will buy a book just to read a chapter or segment of the book that seems most interesting. If anxiety is something that you struggle with regularly, I would advise you to read the book in its entirety, or as much of it as you can. The reason that I make this suggestion is that you will probably learn something about every type of anxiety mentioned in this book if you read all of the chapters. You might even discover a different type of anxiety that is relevant to your situation that you had previously been unaware of. The book will also include journaling prompts and space for you to journal, as you make your way through this book. So, try to read the book in its entirety and complete the journal prompts that seem most appropriate to you. With all of this said, I want to now welcome you to this book. I hope that it will prove to be most enlightening to you and something that you can recommend to other people who struggle with this very common psychological issue.

Chapter One

The Function of Anxiety and How It Can Go Wrong

"I MUST NOT FEAR. FEAR IS THE mind-killer. Fear is the little-death that brings total obliteration..." begins one of the most famous quotes in science fiction, from Frank Herbert's classic novel, *Dune*. Perhaps you can relate to that quote? Fear and anxiety may not be the same exact thing, but they are closely related. There are many among us who *hate* fear and anxiety. As Shakespeare wrote, "Our doubts are traitors, and make us lose the good we oft might win by fearing to attempt." There anxiety is, causing us to lose the good we oft might win! But, if anxiety is so bad, why is it such a powerful aspect of our psychological makeup? Is there really nothing good about feeling anxiety? I invite you to join me, as we explore our complicated relationship with anxiety.

I want to start this journey by asking a question: what is anxiety, at its core, and what purpose does it serve? Before you read on, I want you to spend a minute thinking about this question. What does it mean to be anxious? I have worked with many clients who have struggled with significant anxiety in their lives. I tell them that anxiety is normal, and that everyone feels anxiety about all kinds of things throughout the course of their lives. What separates the clients that end up in a clinic talking to a therapist from an ordinary person concerned with the troubles of everyday life is usually the *degree* of anxiety that they are dealing with, not necessarily the *kind* of anxiety they experience. So, what is anxiety? And why do some people see therapists to help them deal with it?

I have often explained anxiety, as I understand and experience it, as the part of your mind that is trying to keep you alive and safe. When anxiety is functioning well, it is keeping you aware of real threats to your safety and well being. You could call this *functional anxiety*. Of course, just as there is functional anxiety, there is also *dysfunctional anxiety*, which is the similar experience of feeling "on edge" or "uneasy" about something, without the anxiety serving its proper function of keeping you aware and alert to real threats to your safety and well-being. As we go on, let's look at some examples of what I mean by "functional" and "dysfunctional" anxiety.

For *functional anxiety*, I want you to imagine some of the following scenarios: a college student, working on his computer, realizes that he has become distracted by posting on social media and realizes that he only has a few more hours until the deadline to submit his essay for the English class he's taking, which increases his anxiety level, which he resolves by getting back on task and finishing the paper before the deadline; a father worries about whether his child will be able to afford college tuition when they grow up, so he resolves the anxiety by setting aside some money every month to put into a savings account that the child can use later to pay for their college tuition; a woman driving her car begins to notice unusual sounds coming from her car's engine, causing her to feel anxiety about driving, which she resolves by going to the car mechanic. The process is very straightforward: your brain becomes aware of a potential threat or stressor, you begin to feel anxiety, the anxiety is uncomfortable, so you resolve the anxiety by taking action to make whatever changes are necessary.

Dysfunctional anxiety, as the name implies, involves a maladaptive stress response that is experienced by individuals. It does not follow the simple process mentioned above. The anxiety program that runs in your brain can go wrong in a lot of different ways. You might call these "dysfunctional anxiety types." Let's look at a few examples: a person locks themselves up inside their home, unwilling to leave because of their fear and anxiety that something awful will happen if they go out into a public place alone; a young woman's heart begins to race and she is unable to concentrate as she sits in class, when a man that reminds her of someone that had assaulted her takes a seat nearby; a man reports feeling constantly "on edge," unable to sleep well at night and often snapping at loved ones; a person confides in their therapist that they feel terrified when they are away from their romantic partner, worried that the person might leave them or that something bad could happen to that person.

Anxiety Types

You may know someone who has had to deal with something similar to those examples I just listed. Perhaps you have even experienced one of these symptoms at some point in your life. Many people have, as it turns out. The American Psychiatric Association has documented a number of psychological conditions, which we call "disorders," because the symptoms are usually intense enough that they significantly impair a person's ability to function normally and adapt to changes in their life. Let's explore these conditions together, as I explain what types of conditions I have included in this book, what other types of anxiety I believe should be included with them, and what they share in common.

One of the things that just about all forms of dysfunctional anxiety share in common with each other is that they create what's called a "false positive" response. Let me explain. A "false positive" occurs when your mind over-reacts to something (creates too much anxiety) or when it tells you to be anxious about something that isn't really a threat (an irrational fear of something). You see, there are "true positives," "false positives," "true negatives," and "false negatives." In the case of a "true positive," your brain correctly interprets something in your perception as a thing that you should be anxious about, which you can then resolve by addressing it. In the case of a "false positive," we see a threat where there is none or we have an exaggerated anxiety response to something. In the case of a "true negative," your mind correctly identifies that something is not worthy of feeling anxious about (perhaps a house spider or driving your car to work every day). In the case of a "false negative," a person fails to identify something as a threat that truly is a threat (imagine the people who die every year doing risky stunts in exchange for attention on social media).

It's usually the case that we treat people who are dealing with "false positives" of anxiety rather than any of the other types, for a simple reason. In the case of a true positive, our brain is correctly identifying a threat and we deal with it accordingly. In the case of a "false negative," those people typically never complain about the problem until it's too late and something awful happens to them. Anxiety, then, is a gift. While it may make us feel uncomfortable and "ill at ease," it protects us and keeps us safe.

The first anxiety "type" that we will learn about in this book is *Generalized Anxiety*, named after the disorder that it comes from. With this type of anxiety, a person is constantly on edge, unable to quiet their mind, often struggling to sleep well, always worried about something or someone. It's one of the more common diagnoses that therapists treat. The next anxiety type is the broad category of *phobias*, which include quite a number of things. Some examples might include: fear of heights, fear of flying, fear of the dark, fear of being outside one's home in an open space, fear of snakes, fear of spiders, and the list goes on, but you get the idea. Often times, phobias have their basis in something real. You *should* be afraid of being up too high, in certain cases. But when the discomfort is so great that you can't do most of the things that people normally do (like get into an elevator), we have crossed over into the realm of dysfunction.

After we finish with phobias, we will move on to Post Traumatic Stress. Although this section seems like it might only apply to people with PTSD, I feel that it is somewhat applicable to the general population as well. Everyone has trauma of some kind at some point in their lives. It's nearly impossible to go through childhood without having your feelings hurt at some point. As you get older, you have to deal with the death of people you knew and loved. And, of course, traffic accidents can happen. People serve in the military, police force, and fire departments. There are plenty of high stress work environments to go around. So, we will delve into some of the symptoms of PTSD and talk about how to deal with tense moments of high stress and how to overcome past trauma.

Continuing on through the DSM-5, we turn our focus to Social Anxiety Disorder. As the name implies, this disorder is characterized by extreme levels of anxiety that are experienced by individuals when they are in social situations. Although most people experience some degree of anxiety in certain social situations, people who have this disorder tend to have extremely high anxiety levels in nearly all social situations. The primary cause of anxiety in these cases can be an excessive worry about being judged negatively by other people. We will discuss some methods therapists use to help individuals that suffer with this condition.

Panic Disorder is the next topic that we will take on. This disorder is characterized by recurrent panic attacks that can often happen at unexpected or unpredictable times. In this chapter we will look at how panic attacks are experienced and what people can do to help manage the anxiety around not knowing when they will arise. We will also look at ways we can manage a panic attack, if we begin to feel one come on, and we will touch on some of the treatments that are available for people who have this disorder.

Next up, we focus on attachment styles. This is a significant theoretical model within the subfield of psychology that deals with how infants attach to their caregivers. We will only touch on the ideas briefly, but long enough to address an important set of concepts within the field of attachment theory: *Anxious Attachment*. Many people report having symptoms associated with anxious attachment. Primarily, this type of anxiety is thought to result in a parenting style that was a bit too inconsistent, as it relates to the caregiver providing rapid response to the child's needs. When people talk about having "trust issues" or "fear of abandonment," it is generally thought that they are talking about *Anxious Attachment*. Understanding why you feel this way will be important, and we will also discuss how you can address the associated thoughts and feelings when they arise.

Having wrapped up the section on attachment styles, we take a departure from the DSM-5 to tackle a seemingly universal type of anxiety: *existential anxiety*. This has been described by philosophers and psychologists as humanity's struggle with meaning. You may already recognize some of the names associated with this area of literature: Friedrich Nietzsche, Fyodor Dostoevsky, Viktor Frankl, Albert Camus, and more recently Jordan Peterson. Existential psychology and therapy examines man's struggle to resolve some fundamental truths that come with existing as a human. As a human being, we are an embodied mind. We are frail creatures subjected to the forces of nature, particularly aging and death. As such, death and suffering are a fundamental aspect of our existence. The limited nature of our bodies and our lives forces us to grapple with how to spend our limited time and how to find meaning in a seemingly meaningless world.

Although *Substance Use Disorder* is not considered an anxiety disorder, I have chosen to address this topic, as it is very relevant to the topic of anxiety. In particular, the use of alcohol as a way to ameliorate symptoms of extreme anxiety is a very well known phenomenon to psychotherapists. However, alcohol is by no means the only substance that is used or abused by people looking to escape the pain and suffering that constant dysfunctional anxiety brings. I wanted to address this issue from several different angles. I'd like to explore what kind of relationship we should have with the substances we are putting into our body. I would also like to address any hidden beliefs we might have about people who use substances to address their anxiety symptoms. Part of this section will be devoted to transitioning into alternative interventions that a person can use to achieve the same effects as substances, in terms of symptom alleviation.

Finally, you will notice that I've included a few chapters in this book that aren't specifically about "anxiety types," but that are very relevant in a discussion about anxiety types. In particular, the sections about the anxieties of modern living, substance use, and sticking points are essential elements of a book designed to address anxiety and for equipping the reader with useful tools for resolving anxiety in a functionally appropriate way. I believe that addressing the aspects of modern living that contribute significantly to our feelings of anxiety is important, because it sets the stage upon which our lives are acted out. If you think about it, much of our anxiety comes from environmental cues. As for "sticking points," the reason that I have included this section is that, in my work with clients who have struggled with anxiety issues, I have often noticed that the clients would sometimes come to a point in their work where they would show up, session after session, and not have anything new to report. They seemed "stuck," not having taken any meaningful action on the problem that they were dealing with. I wanted to include a section on how to avoid sticking points and what to do if you should find yourself feeling "stuck."

Considerations As You Continue

I feel that I should address some issues and provide some disclaimers before we get into the meat of this book. The point may seem obvious, but I will make note of it regardless: talking about the topic of anxiety and the various types of anxiety might provoke or trigger your own anxiety. Some of the topics that we cover in this book might strike a person as being a bit "dark" in tone. In particular, I'm talking about the section on *Existential Anxiety*. Although I've talked about this issue, thought about this issue, wrestled with this issue enough in my life to the point where the concepts are no longer scary or threatening, I recognize that not everyone has been exposed to these concepts to the same degree and thus a person could have a very strong emotional reaction to the kind of concepts that we will be dealing with in that chapter. Also, when we're talking about post traumatic stress, you might find yourself re-living past events in your life that are potentially terrifying. So, consider yourself warned as you go forward. This book may bring up some very real, very unpleasant feelings. That's how you know you're doing real work.

Next, I would advise you not to necessarily think of these anxiety disorders as "all or none." Even with people who suffer from these disorders, they may go through periods of remission, where they don't feel the symptoms to the degree necessary for a clinical diagnosis. Similarly, someone who doesn't cross the threshold necessary to meet a clinical diagnosis might still have to deal with anxiety levels that are above what might be thought of as "normal" or "average." For such a person, the tools and interventions mentioned in this book might be helpful in bringing their anxiety down to a more comfortable level and may help them develop a more healthy relationship with their anxiety.

There is one final thing that I would like to mention, at the close of this chapter. I have written this book to be thorough and thought provoking, as it relates to the subject of anxiety. However, I do want to caution you against the dangers of rumination. What I mean by this is that there is a danger in thinking that, just because you read a bunch of books about anxiety or you see a therapist about your anxiety, you are solving your anxiety problem. The truth is that while these things certainly *can* be instrumental steps on your journey towards growth and resolving your anxiety in a functional way, it doesn't mean that the thing that you are feeling anxious about will go away. Talking about your problems can feel cathartic and it might make you feel good to have someone listen to your problems. However, the problem begins to arise when you re-hash your problems and anxieties over and over again without taking any meaningful action. Remember that the purpose of anxiety is to prod us out of our complacency so that we take action. When we re-hash our anxieties over and over without taking meaningful action, we run the risk of *increasing* our anxiety levels. The next chapter will explore how to face anxiety in an effective and functional way.

Chapter Two

A Toolbox for Defeating Dysfunctional Anxiety

WELCOME TO CHAPTER TWO! I have prepared what I feel is an extensive list of tools that are the most effective treatments for people that deal with an oppressive level of anxiety. The reason that I am putting this chapter at the front of the book is that I don't want people to have to read through hundreds of pages of material before they finally get to something that can be of use to them. I want to deliver the good stuff to you as soon as possible. Also, as promised, here is the pass code for the Facebook group associated with this book: **4292025**. You don't have to join this group, but it's my desire to create spaces and communities where people can meet to solve problems and talk about what has been helpful for them in their lives. I believe very strongly in the importance of community. I will also be creating a YouTube channel associated with this book as well, which I will periodically post helpful information on.

Cognitive Behavior Therapy

Any book written on the topic of anxiety would be incomplete without a section devoted to Cognitive Behavior Therapy (often referred to as CBT). CBT is considered among mental health care workers to be the "gold standard" for treatment with individuals suffering from anxiety and depression. There are a number of reasons that it has earned this level of respect in the Healthcare system. It just works. The ideas have been around for decades, and there is a sports stadium full of clinical studies that have been done in which CBT was used as a treatment. The essence of CBT is that it trains individuals to think more critically about some of the beliefs and assumptions that become automatic thoughts for people that suffer from anxiety and depression. The name may sound strange, but it basically just means "thought behavior." If we change our thoughts, we change our feelings. But more on that later.

Cognitive Behavior Therapy works best when you have ample time to sit down and rationally reflect on your thoughts. You have to be very intentional about how you approach the process. The CBT process doesn't happen by accident. It also takes some degree of intelligence and introspection to be able to do it properly. I have had clients that might have benefited from CBT interventions, but their capacity for abstract thinking simply wasn't developed enough to have the types of conversations needed for CBT. Sadly, a number of clients that walk through the doors of the clinic have some kind of cognitive impairment that creates a lot of the problems that they are experiencing. However, the good news is that if you are reading this book right now you probably have the cognitive capacity to understand the concepts in CBT and to apply them to your life.

At the heart of CBT is the core concept of the A-B-C theory of emotions. The concept goes like this: first we have an activating event in our lives (**A**), which we interpret through a mental filtering process that interprets the event and creates some kind of meaning from it based on our beliefs (**B**), and the result of these beliefs and assumptions is the resulting emotional output, or consequence (**C**). So, some event happens to you, your brain forms a judgment of the event, and based on that judgment you feel some kind of emotion about the event. We call that the A-B-C theory of emotion, developed by Albert Ellis.

Let's look at one real life example. Back before I had been exposed to psychotherapy models, I was a very anxious and insecure young man. At one point, I called a female friend of mine from High School. I heard that she had broken up with her boyfriend, and now it was my shot. So, I called her and asked her out. She told me that, "I won't be available on that date. I'm going on a trip with my family. But when I get back, you should call me again." I told her that I would, and I hung up the phone. I was very disappointed. It was so difficult for me to work up the courage to ask a girl out, back then. "She's just being nice," I told myself. "She wanted a way to turn me down without having to turn me down." "What a fool I've made of myself." These were the thoughts that I kept telling myself. And you know what? I never did call her back or ask her out again. It was the sad end of a friendship, as well, because I was too insecure to keep in touch with her or include her in my life after that. I use this as an example of how negative thoughts can, at the very least, limit your opportunities in life and amplify your anxiety.

Sometimes I wonder how many other people in this world have done something similarly foolish because they let their emotions run the show and don't bother to use that amazing prefrontal cortex that we humans have been given that allows us to think rationally. So, where did things go wrong in that scenario, and how could they have turned out differently? Using the A-B-C theory of emotions, we can hypothesize that my belief about what the girl had told me was causing me to feel anxiety and discouragement. As you can see, there are many interpretations about the activating event, which for me was being told, "no, I can't meet you that day." As we will see later, taking a more critical approach to our thoughts and beliefs could have led me to question the assumption that she was only telling me the other part just to let me down easy. Here's one potential CBT intervention: "okay, let's assume that there's a 90% chance that she was just letting me down easy, but there could also potentially be a 10% chance that she's genuinely going to be out of town with her family and does want you to call her back again when she gets back. That still leaves plenty of room for you to end up going on a date with this girl that you like." Another approach would be to ask, "why would a girl that you have never known to be duplicitous or deceitful suddenly lie to you, only to find herself in the same situation of having to say 'no' to you again at a later date?" That is an example of simply following the logic of the idea in question to its rational conclusion. The take-away for these examples is that we are using a logical reasoning process to address the automatic thinking that affects your emotional state, so that you can bring your emotions into alignment with rational thought.

Most of CBT's interventions and tools are designed for just that: to aid you in making more rational decisions and dealing with the negative emotions that arise from those irrational thoughts. A lot of the core concepts in CBT deal with "cognitive distortions," or distorted beliefs. Let's review some of them. The first is *all or none thinking:* viewing situations in black-and-white terms, with no middle ground. For example, thinking "If I'm not perfect, I'm a failure." For clarification, it's not that there can never be any beliefs that are all-or-none, it's just that some of our all or none thinking can get us into trouble. Elvis Presley is either dead or alive. That's all or none. But believing that if you don't get into your first choice of college you will be unhappy for the rest of your life might be an all or none assumption that could potentially contribute to your unnecessary burden of anxiety or depression.

Another thing that people often do is what CBT theory calls *overgeneralization*, which is where a person makes broad conclusions based on a single incident. For instance, concluding that because one job interview went poorly, all future interviews will be failed attempts. There's also the concept of *discounting the positive*, which is what a lot of depressed people do. This is where people believe that positive experiences or achievements don't count for some reason. For example, someone might say, "That compliment doesn't mean anything because they were just being nice." Here's another idea that we've all probably been guilty of, at some point: *jumping to conclusions*. This is where a person makes assumptions without supporting evidence. This includes *mind reading* (believing you know what others are thinking) and *future predicting* (predicting a future that you don't know).

One concept in CBT that I really like and found that my clients often can relate to is the concept of *catastrophizing*, which is where a person imagines the worst-case scenario or believes that a situation will have disastrous consequences. This often leads to heightened anxiety about the outcome. I also call this phenomenon *doom spiraling*. I will give you an example. "My girlfriend broke up with me. That must mean that I'm not attractive to women or I can't keep them attracted to me. And if I can't keep a woman interested, then that means I will never have a wife or family. If I can't have a wife and a family, then I will just be alone forever. If I'm alone forever, I'll just be unhappy for my whole life and die alone." You go from one small incident to a world-ending catastrophe! I remember explaining this concept to one of my clients and he smiled knowingly at me. "That's exactly what I do," he said. Sadly, he's not alone.

CBT therapists also describe something called *emotional reasoning*, which is where a person assumes that feelings reflect reality. For instance, "I feel anxious about this presentation, so it must mean I will mess it up." The next concept is something that a lot of people do. I view it as a type of overgeneralization, which we covered previously. It is called *labeling and mislabeling*. This is where we
assign negative labels to oneself or others based on mistakes or behaviors. For instance, labeling oneself as a "loser" after a setback. The last concept that I am going to cover is called *personalization*. This is where an individual takes responsibility for events outside

of one's control or blames oneself for negative outcomes. For example, thinking, "It's my fault that my friend is upset," even when it's unrelated.

As you can see, CBT heavily emphasizes the importance of rational, logical thinking because when we are experiencing crippling levels of anxiety, it is often due to a distortion in our thinking. CBT therapists will often use thought experiments and exercises to help clients realign their thoughts with reality. Let's look at a quick example. In particular, people who suffer from phobias often over-estimate the likelihood of an adverse event occurring. For example, for someone who has a fear of flying, a CBT therapist might take them through a *risk analysis and management* exercise. They might ask the client to estimate the likelihood of being in a fatal plane accident. After the client gives their estimation, the two would look up the actual probability of being in a fatal plane accident. Then the client and therapist might identify and evaluate the factors that could influence the risk. They would then work together to reduce or manage the risk. Finally, the counselor would discuss the inevitable risk and uncertainty inherent in life. The therapist might point out that if a person wants to be active and influential in the world, one has to accept a certain degree of risk associated with performing numerous low-risk activities, such as driving to work, or taking public transportation to work, going to the store, etc.

Another common exercise that CBT therapists often utilize with their clients is what's called a *cost/benefit analysis*. With this exercise, the aim is to consciously identify the discrete benefits and costs associated with acting on or entertaining certain beliefs. In the case of a fear of flying, the therapist might point out the real benefits of never flying. After all, when you fly there is always some kind of minimal risk that you are running of some kind of catastrophic event occurring, which may result in your death. So, the benefit of never traveling by airline might be preventing one's own death in the extremely improbable event of a catastrophe. However, the therapist might point out that the cost associated with never traveling by airline might be longer transit time by an alternative transport method that may be even more dangerous, such as when traveling by car.

I am going to include some worksheets with this section, so that you can always refer back to them, when needed. You can also search google for "CBT worksheets" if you want maybe a slightly different take on the idea. All of these worksheets are generally designed to help you through the process of *cognitive restructuring*: identifying unhelpful or limiting beliefs, deconstructing them, and replacing them with a new, more helpful thought/ belief.

Personally, I have found CBT ideas to be very helpful, for both myself and clients that I have worked with in the clinic. It works particularly well with people who are of average to above average intelligence. It also tends to work well if the person is naturally self-reflective and has a good amount of self-awareness. I would also say that it works better with people who have lower levels of symptom severity than those with a very high degree of symptom severity. In terms of anxiety types, I would say that people who deal with Generalized Anxiety will tend to do better with CBT interventions compared to other anxiety types. However, CBT is a good tool for dealing with anxiety, in general.

I want to make a final side note about CBT. There are people out there in the world that think CBT amounts to "think happy thoughts" to make your psychological problems go away. This is an incredibly ignorant understanding of the model. We are not just trying to put a smiley face on everything in order to feel better. Rather, we are attempting to monitor our thoughts, as we begin to feel anxious, in order to understand what is making us feel that way, and then we analyze those thoughts to see if they have merit to them. If we determine that there is something that we should legitimately be concerned about, we adjust our thoughts and behaviors to address those concerns. If, however, our anxiety seems to be based on irrational presuppositions, then we must confront those illogical beliefs and replace them with ones that are more functional and rational.

The A-B-C Worksheet

The purpose of this worksheet is to teach you how to use the A-B-C method to analyze and restructure thinking patterns.

Activating event (was there a precipitating event that brought on these thoughts?):

Beliefs about the event:	Replacement belief:
Feelings/ Emotions:	Feelings/ Emotions:

Cost/Benefit Analysis Worksheet

The purpose of this worksheet is to teach you how to use the concept of cost/benefit analysis to apply to beliefs or behaviors.

Describe the current belief under investigation:

Benefits- what benefits does having this belief or behavior give to you?	Costs- what opportunities or possibilities are you potentially missing out on?

Analysis- are you happy with this trade off?

Risk Analysis and Management Worksheet

The purpose of this worksheet is to teach you how to analyze the risk of an unwanted event occurring in your life, and deciding how best to minimize that risk.

1) Identify and define the risk:

"I fear that if I go outside, I might have a panic attack and collapse."

2) Assess the actual probability and severity:

"How many times in the past year have I actually fainted or had a panic attack outside?"

3) Identify and evaluate the factors that could influence the risk:

"Wearing comfortable shoes and avoiding extreme heat reduce the risk of fainting."

4) Develop strategies to reduce or manage the risk:

"I will plan short outings with a trusted friend while holding a calming object."

5) Establish a monitoring and review system:

"I will keep a journal of experiences when facing feared situations, noting the actual outcomes versus expected outcomes."

6) Accept uncertainty and limitations:

"I accept that no safety measure can eliminate all risk—uncertainty is inherent in life. The goal is not to eliminate risk entirely but to manage it effectively and accept that some level of uncertainty is part of normal life."

Behavioral Therapy

The next tool that I want to introduce to you is from what is known as "the school of Behaviorism." From this branch of psychology we get a lot of different techniques that are used in various applications of psychotherapy. The school of Behaviorism owes its origins to the work of Ivan Pavlov. Perhaps you are already aware of the story of Ivan and his salivating dogs? What Ivan discovered was later formalized into a theory of learning called "classical conditioning." However, the idea that we will be looking at here is called "exposure therapy."

Exposure therapy is a psychological treatment widely used to reduce fear and anxiety associated with specific phobias, obsessive-compulsive disorder, post-traumatic stress disorder, and other anxiety-related conditions. Its core principle is straightforward: gradually and systematically exposing individuals to the feared object, situation, or memory in a safe and controlled way to diminish the power of their anxiety response over time.

At its essence, exposure therapy operates on the idea of *habituation*—the process by which repeated exposure to a feared stimulus leads to a decrease in emotional response. Initially, individuals may experience intense anxiety, but with repeated exposure, their nervous system gradually learns that the stimulus is not as threatening as perceived. As this process unfolds, their fear diminishes, and they develop greater tolerance and confidence in facing similar situations.

The process typically begins with *assessment and preparation,* where the therapist works with the individual to identify their specific fears and create an *exposure hierarchy*—a ranked list of feared stimuli or situations from least to most anxiety-provoking. The individual then starts exposure at the lower end of this hierarchy, engaging with the feared stimulus in a controlled and safe setting, sometimes through imagination, visualization, or direct confrontation.

A common approach is *systematic, gradual exposure*—for example, someone with a fear of dogs might start by looking at pictures of dogs, then observing a dog from a distance, and eventually gradually approaching or petting a dog. Throughout the process, the therapist encourages the person to remain engaged with the experience, practice relaxation techniques, and observe their anxiety without avoiding or battling it.

The key to the success of exposure therapy is *consistency and repetition*. Over multiple sessions, as the individual encounters the feared stimuli and notices their anxiety decreasing, they build confidence and resistance to fear flare-ups. Importantly, the goal is not to eliminate all anxiety but to reduce its intensity and prevent avoidance behaviors that reinforce the phobia.

The way that you can apply this in your own life is to find a good therapist that will help you through the process, or to attempt to do the process yourself. If you choose to go through the process yourself, I would recommend that you find a friend or family member that can join you in this endeavor. Pick someone who can push you and also provide you with the emotional support necessary as you are putting in the work. Always begin with a stimulus that will activate some degree of anxiety that feels just a little unpleasant to you. You want to shoot for the sweet spot between feeling overwhelmed versus nothing at all. If you choose a stimulus that provokes too much anxiety, then you are actually *sensitizing* yourself more to the feared stimulus. Instead, we are shooting for gradual *desensitization*.

This type of therapy, when paired with CBT cognitive restructuring techniques, often makes a powerful duo. You are reprogramming your mind at the same time you are reprogramming your body to respond to your anxiety in a new way. As you will see, we can pile other techniques on top of each other, as well. For example, you might use some pharmaceutical prescriptions to help deal with intense anxiety reactions during the process of desensitization.

In general, I tend to think that *exposure therapy* works best with anxiety types like *post traumatic stress disorder* and the various phobias, but it is also used with many of the other anxiety types as well, including: *social anxiety disorder*, *panic disorder*, and *generalized anxiety disorder*. Remember that the key to exposure therapy is to take small, manageable steps. Do you recall that quote from Frank Herbert's novel, *Dune*? The full quote makes reference to facing one's fear. This is what we are doing with exposure therapy: making you face your fear, one manageable step at a time.

Pharmaceutical Treatment

There are a number of different pharmaceutical treatment options available to people who suffer from severe anxiety symptoms. The psychological community in general has a very awkward relationship with drug therapies. On the one hand, therapists and counselors want to solve the underlying psychological problems in their clients' lives. They would like the client to gain insights and build skills that lead to psychological resiliency as a result of their work together, rather than just taking a pill. Also, there is the issue of clients potentially becoming addicted to their medication or suffering from some kind of unwanted side effect. On the other hand, there is no denying that prescription drugs for anxiety, when managed well, can lead to significant reduction in severe anxiety symptoms for their clients.

The general consensus at the time I was making my way through graduate school was that the best practice for treating anxiety disorders was to begin treatment with an appropriate dosage of medications that could decrease the short-term symptom intensity. While the client was developing new skills and working their way through therapy, they would slowly begin to decrease the dosage of their medication, until they had worked their way entirely off of the meds and were managing the anxiety on their own. This is, of course, in the best possible scenario. Some clients might need to stay on anxiety medications for a very long time or perhaps indefinitely, if they want to reduce their anxiety symptoms. In any case, I will not advise anyone on which medication that they should take for their symptoms. I think that is a conversation that you should have with your physician, your med manager, or your psychiatrist. However, I will provide you with a summary of what prescription drugs are currently available and what they do. Keep in mind that prescription meds can sometimes create unwanted side-effects.

Pharmaceutical treatment of anxiety disorders involves a diverse range of medications targeting various neurochemical pathways to alleviate symptoms and improve functioning. The most commonly prescribed are *Selective Serotonin Reuptake Inhibitors (SSRIs)* and *Serotonin-Norepinephrine Reuptake Inhibitors (SNRIs)*, which are considered first-line treatments due to their proven effectiveness and favorable safety profiles. SSRIs, such as **fluoxetine**, **sertraline**, and **escitalopram**, work by increasing serotonin levels in the brain, helping to regulate mood and anxiety. SNRIs, like **venlafaxine** and **duloxetine**, increase both serotonin and norepinephrine, which can be particularly beneficial in cases where SSRIs are ineffective.

Buspirone is a unique anti-anxiety medication that acts as a partial agonist at serotonin receptors, providing a non-sedative and non-addictive option primarily used for *generalized anxiety disorder*. It's valued for its safety in long-term use, although it requires several weeks for full effectiveness.

Benzodiazepines, including **diazepam**, **lorazepam**, and **alprazolam**, offer rapid relief of acute anxiety symptoms by enhancing the neurotransmitter GABA (gamma-aminobutyric acid) activity. GABA functions as the brain's primary inhibitory neurotransmitter. Despite their effectiveness, benzodiazepines are typically used short-term because they can lead to dependence, tolerance, and cognitive impairment if used excessively or over extended periods.

Tricyclic antidepressants (TCAs) such as **imipramine** and **clomipramine**, as well as *Monoamine Oxidase Inhibitors (MAOIs)* like **phenelzine**, are older classes of medications. They are generally reserved for treatment-resistant cases due to their broader side effect profiles, including risks of weight gain, dry mouth, and hypertensive crises with MAOIs.

Beta-blockers such as **propranolol** are effective for situational or performance anxiety by blocking adrenaline effects, thus reducing physical symptoms like rapid heartbeat and trembling during anxiety-provoking events.

Finally, **pregabalin** and **hydroxyzine** are occasionally used as adjuncts or alternatives — pregabalin for generalized anxiety, especially when other medications are unsuitable, and hydroxyzine for short-term relief due to its sedative effects.

Existential Therapy

Recall from chapter one that *existential anxiety* refers to the type of anxiety that is specific to life as a human being. Although there is no one universally agreed upon definition for existential anxiety, it typically refers to the reality of living as an embodied mind, and everything that comes with it. Typically, literature that touches on things like being thrown into life/ existence with no real instruction guide or knowledge about life's inherent meaning, the finite nature of life, the limitations of living in a frail body that degrades over time, and the general struggle to find meaning in one's day to day actions, is typically thought to be existentialist literature.

To give you a sense for a client that might be struggling with existential anxiety symptoms, consider a fictional case study. A man comes into therapy complaining of feeling bored, frustrated, and lost in his current life. He's married with two children. However, as the days go bye, he feels less and less connected to his family. He dislikes his job, which he feels no real passion or motivation to go to work at every day. Worst yet, he feels that he is no longer in love with his wife or children, who he feels are becoming more and more distant from him every day. Secretly, he dreams of running off with his female coworker that is 15 years younger than him. This is because his coworker reminds him of when he was young and full of life.

That fictional case study, similar to the character of Lester Burnham in the movie *American Beauty*, is a kind of cliché of men going through a "midlife crisis." Existential psychologists would say that this kind of crisis develops for a variety of reasons associated with the psychological pressures that come from existential anxiety. As an example, an existential psychologist might choose to focus specifically on the theme of feeling frustrated at work, and that there is no deeper meaning to the work besides collecting a paycheck. Existential therapy might also focus on the feelings of anxiety and dread experienced by the client associated with growing older and knowing that death looms larger with every passing year. Perhaps part of the attraction with the younger work colleague is due to the feelings of youth and memories of a time when they weren't burdened by a growing sense of dread at the idea of one's finite life span?

What defines existential therapy as its own genre of therapy is owing to the themes that it focuses on. Although there may be other brands of existential therapy, the one that I am most familiar with is Viktor Frankl's *Logotherapy*. Frankl developed and formalized many of the ideas of logotherapy while he was a prisoner in the Nazi concentration camps of Auschwitz and Dachau. Let's look at Frankl's conceptualization of the primary paths to meaning and then we will look at some techniques that we might take and apply to our lives to address existential anxiety.

The first pathway to meaning that Frankl espouses is through *creative values*. Creative values refer to what individuals give to the world through their contributions and achievements. This path to meaning emphasizes active engagement in tasks and roles that individuals find fulfilling and purposeful. It could involve creating art, developing a project, contributing to a community, or nurturing personal and professional relationships. In the realm of creative values, work takes on a significant role. However, it's important to note that it's not just any work but work that aligns with one's values and aspirations that contributes to a sense of purpose. For example, an artist might find profound meaning in their paintings, while a teacher might see it in shaping the minds of students. Frankl posits that when individuals apply themselves creatively, they transcend the mundane aspects of life, channeling their efforts into something that outlasts them, contributing to their sense of legacy.

The second pathway that Frankl discusses is *experiential values*. This path emphasizes the importance of fully experiencing life and the world. Experiential values highlight appreciation for beauty, love, culture, nature, and the range of experiences life offers. It's about what we take from the world emotionally and spiritually. Love is singled out as a primary experiential value because it allows individuals to see the uniqueness and intrinsic value of others. Through loving relationships, people find meaning by deeply connecting with others, understanding, and appreciating them. Experiencing beauty and wonder in art, music, or nature also provides fulfilling meaning. These experiences can evoke feelings of awe and connection to something greater, something beyond oneself that resonates with one's inner values and beliefs.

The third path to meaning for Viktor Frankl is *attitudinal values*. Attitudinal values involve the choices and attitudes individuals adopt, particularly when faced with difficult situations, such as suffering, loss, or adversity. According to Frankl, while we cannot always control our circumstances, we can control our responses. Frankl's own experience in concentration camps exemplifies this path, as he found meaning in the midst of suffering by choosing his attitude toward his circumstances. His stance was that suffering itself doesn't add meaning, but rather the attitude taken toward suffering can. Central to this path is the concept of seeing suffering as an opportunity for personal growth or as a means to achieve a bigger purpose. It involves courage and resilience, transforming tragic circumstances into opportunities to develop the human spirit.

Now let's shift our attention to the first technique that Frankl uses and which you can utilize in your own life to help you resolve or reduce your anxiety. First is *dereflection*, which involves redirecting the focus away from oneself and toward others or specific tasks. It's particularly useful for individuals who may have become self-absorbed or fixated on certain issues, leading to anxiety or obsessive behaviors. By engaging in meaningful tasks or focusing on external factors, a person can break the cycle of self-preoccupation. For instance, a person dealing with social anxiety might be guided to shift their focus from worrying about how they are perceived, to genuinely paying attention to what others are saying and feeling.

The second technique Frankl would use in logotherapy would be the use of *paradoxical intention*. This technique employs humor and irony to help individuals confront their fears and anxieties. By encouraging clients to intentionally exaggerate their anxious symptoms or fears humorously, the emotional response is often diminished. For example, someone with insomnia might be instructed to try to stay awake as long as possible, or a person who fears blushing in public might be encouraged to try to blush on purpose. This reversal in approach can reduce the power of anticipatory anxiety and facilitate coping.

The third technique from logotherapy that Frankl would likely use is *Socratic dialogue*. Named after the Greek philosopher Socrates, this technique involves guided questioning to help clients uncover their beliefs and values. Through a dialogue that explores personal thoughts and assumptions, individuals can gain insight and clarity regarding what truly matters to them. Socratic dialogue is a collaborative process where the therapist aids clients in examining their life goals, choices, and attitudes, helping them recognize self-imposed limitations and discover pathways to authentic living. Think of Socratic dialogue as a series of open-ended questions meant to probe deeper thinking, similar to CBT. For instance, "when do you find yourself not feeling a sense of overwhelming anxiety?" Or "after which activities, if any, do you feel the anxiety begin to significantly decrease in intensity?"

Logotherapy's techniques are synergistic, each reinforcing the other to empower individuals to embrace life with a sense of purpose and resilience. At its core, Logotherapy offers a roadmap for navigating the existential vacuum—a sense of emptiness or meaninglessness—by encouraging personal responsibility, freedom, and the relentless search for meaning. We will discuss this topic more deeply in the chapter dedicated to existentialism.

Physiological Interventions

I think that it's important, at the outset of this section, to clarify what I mean by "physiological interventions," since you could argue that every psychological intervention has some kind of effect on a person's physiology. Also, medications will most definitely produce an affect on a person's physiology as well. However, I thought that it was necessary to distinguish medications from the kinds of physiological interventions that we will talk about in this section. When I talk about "physiological interventions," I'm generally talking about the non-conscious bodily processes that contribute to your overall psychological state. The goal, with this section, is to be able to recognize your internal emotional state and have more control. When I was young, I was driven more by anxiety and I was constantly worried about myself and how I was being perceived by others. Now, in my 40s, I have almost the opposite issue. I generally have very good control of my anxiety. I am able to constantly question what feelings are based on the assumptions that I'm making. Sometimes, I now face the challenge of having to work myself into a higher state of anxiety, so that I can be motivated enough to be productive or solve some problem that I need to deal with. By learning some of the following skills, I hope to give you more ownership of your anxiety so you can use it appropriately in your life.

Nutrition and exercise are two of the most important physiological factors, as it relates to mood and one's anxiety state. I'm sure that you have all had the experience of being "hangry" at some point in your life. I use that as an example of how your mood can swing throughout your day based on your food intake. I'm not a certified nutritionist, but I can tell you that balancing your amount of calorie intake (eating approximately as many calories as you expend in a day) and trying to keep your calories evenly distributed throughout the day can do wonders for your overall mood and sense of well-being. Also, it should be noted that you need to watch your caffeine intake. Some level of caffeine is probably fine. I, myself, drink coffee about every other day. However, large amounts of caffeine intake can result in increased heart rate, palpitations, high blood pressure, insomnia, anxiety, jitters, upset stomach, nausea, and headaches.

Exercise has been widely recognized for its positive effects on mental wellness, including its ability to alleviate symptoms of anxiety and improve overall mental health. Engaging in regular physical activity can lead to significant psychological benefits due to its impact on various physiological and biochemical processes. Regular physical activity also encourages the growth of new neurons in specific areas of the brain, such as the hippocampus, which is involved in mood regulation and memory. This process, known as neurogenesis, has been linked to improved emotional resilience and cognitive function, further contributing to mental wellness (Hamer, M., & Chida, Y., 2008).

In terms of anxiety, exercise has been shown to provide both short-term and long-term benefits. In the short term, a single session of moderate to vigorous exercise can reduce anxiety levels, providing some immediate relief from symptoms (Petruzzello et al., 1991). Over the long term, engaging in regular exercise can decrease the overall severity of anxiety symptoms and reduce the likelihood of developing anxiety disorders. This is achieved through improved stress response systems and increased self-efficacy and confidence, resulting from mastering physical challenges during exercise (Wipfli, et al., 2008).

Furthermore, physical activity can serve as a valuable distraction from stressors, offering a break from negative thought patterns that often magnify anxiety. Group activities or exercise classes provide social interaction, which can enhance mood and reduce feelings of isolation. Regular exercise is a powerful tool for enhancing mental wellness and managing anxiety. Through a combination of biochemical processes and psychosocial benefits, exercise can significantly contribute to improved mental health outcomes. As research continues to support its efficacy, exercise remains a cornerstone recommendation for individuals seeking to enhance their mental well-being.

Breathing exercises are often used to create a calming effect and decrease anxiety. These exercises can help manage short term periods of high anxiety and, when practiced regularly, contribute to long-term anxiety reduction. One of the most widely used breathing exercises is *Diaphragmatic Breathing* (also known as abdominal or deep breathing). This technique involves fully engaging the diaphragm, allowing for deep inhalation and slow exhalation, promoting a sense of calm. Here's how to practice it: 1) sit or lie down in a comfortable position, 2) place one hand on your chest and one on your abdomen, 3) inhale slowly through your nose, allowing your abdomen to expand while keeping your chest as still as possible, 4) exhale slowly through your mouth, letting your abdomen fall, 5) aim to take longer exhales than inhales, for example, inhaling for four seconds and exhaling for six.

Box breathing, another effective technique, is particularly useful in stressful situations. This method focuses on equal phases of breathing to stabilize the heart rate and reduce stress levels: 1) inhale deeply through your nose for a count of four, 2) hold your breath for a count of four, 3) exhale slowly through your mouth for a count of four, 4) hold your breath again for a count of four before repeating this process.

The next technique, called *4-7-8 breathing* is designed to bring the body into a state of deep relaxation and helps manage anxiety by focusing on rhythm and control: 1) exhale completely through your mouth, 2) inhale quietly through your nose for a count of four, 3) hold your breath for a count of seven, 4) exhale completely through your mouth for a count of eight, 5) repeat the cycle three to four times.

These breathing techniques work by activating the parasympathetic nervous system, which counters the "fight or flight" response induced by anxiety, helping lower heart rate, reduce muscle tension, and promote feelings of relaxation.

Meditation is also an exercise that psychologists have investigated for its ability to attenuate severe anxiety symptoms. Rooted in various ancient traditions, meditation offers numerous mental health benefits, particularly in alleviating symptoms of elevated anxiety. By fostering a state of mindful awareness and promoting a sense of calm, meditation can effectively counter the stress response and enhance emotional well-being. One of the primary benefits of meditation is its ability to reduce anxiety by shifting focus from anxious thoughts to the present moment. This mindfulness aspect helps break the cycle of worry and overthinking, which is a common issue for individuals suffering from severe anxiety. Regular meditation has been shown to decrease levels of cortisol, the stress hormone, thereby reducing physical symptoms of anxiety such as increased heart rate and muscle tension (Goyal et al., 2014).

Moreover, meditation encourages the cultivation of a non-judgmental attitude toward thoughts and feelings, allowing individuals to observe their experiences without being overwhelmed. This can lead to improved emotional regulation and increased resilience in stressful situations. To use meditation to attenuate anxiety, follow these simple steps: 1) find a quiet space- choose a comfortable and quiet environment where you won't be disturbed; 2) posture and breathing- sit or lie down in a relaxed position. Close your eyes gently and begin by taking a few deep breaths to settle into the practice; 3) focus on breath- direct your attention to your breathing. Notice the sensations of inhaling and exhaling. When your mind wanders, gently bring your focus back to your breath; 4) practice mindfulness- allow thoughts to come and go without judgment. Acknowledge them and then return to your focus on the present moment.

Consistency is key, with the use of meditation. Commit to regular practice, even if it's just a few minutes daily. Gradually increase the duration as you become more comfortable. Through consistent practice, meditation can significantly reduce anxiety, enhance mindfulness, and promote overall mental clarity and peace, providing a valuable tool for managing anxiety over the long term.

Journaling is a versatile self-help tool that offers significant psychological benefits, particularly in reducing symptoms of elevated anxiety. By providing a structured way to express thoughts and emotions, journaling facilitates emotional processing and promotes mental clarity.

One of the key benefits of journaling is its ability to help individuals organize and articulate their thoughts and feelings, which can often feel overwhelming when anxious. This process not only aids in understanding the root causes of anxiety but also enables individuals to identify patterns and triggers that exacerbate their symptoms. Research suggests that expressive writing can reduce anxiety levels, enhance mood, and improve overall psychological well-being (Pennebaker & Chung, 2007).

Journaling can also serve as a mindfulness practice, bringing attention to the present moment and creating a sense of distance from stressful thoughts. It encourages self-reflection, fostering a deeper awareness of emotional responses and promoting effective coping strategies. To use journaling to attenuate anxiety, consider these steps: 1) set a regular schedule- dedicate a specific time each day for journaling, creating a consistent routine; 2) create a safe environment- choose a quiet space where you feel comfortable entertaining and expressing your thoughts; 3) write freely- begin by writing about your day, thoughts, or any specific events that have caused anxiety. Don't worry about grammar or coherence; 4) reflect on your feelings- this may be a good time to practice some of those CBT exercises and ideas from earlier in this chapter; 5) identify patterns- over time, review your entries to identify patterns or recurring themes that might require further attention or action.

Sufficient sleep is an absolutely essential element in psychological and emotional well-being. Sleep disruption is one of the most common factors shared between individuals suffering from some form of psychological disorder. If you are not currently sleeping well, you need to begin prioritizing your sleep. Here are some suggestions that may help you to develop a stable, healthy sleeping pattern: try to schedule for approximately 7-9 hours a night; keep your phone out of reach when you go to bed, so that you aren't tempted to get on it and stimulate your brain instead of sleeping; consider engaging in a calming activity before bed; try not to consume foods, beverages, and supplements containing caffeine (i.e. coffee, tea, sodas, chocolate) late in the evening; try to avoid naps and sleeping in on weekends, keep your sleep schedule as consistent as possible.

Final Thoughts

I realize that this list of items gives you a lot to chew on. Each of these tools for therapy will require significant amounts of work to implement on their own. Nutrition and exercise themselves represent significant commitments of time and energy. The CBT skills will take time and practice to develop, as well. Just be patient with yourself and take these skills one step at a time. We will talk about this subject more in the "sticking points" chapter, but I want to tell you right now that there's no need to rush the process. Maybe you could pick one of the previously mentioned interventions to work on every week. Figure out what you can handle and don't overload yourself.

And now, I'd like to provide you with some journaling prompts, as I had mentioned previously. These prompts are intended to help you develop a new habit of calmly reflecting on things that you have been thinking about throughout the day. I think that you will find it to be a very relaxing technique. Sometimes, in my work with clients at the clinic, I would instruct them to spend a few minutes journaling about something. In those sessions, I would typically put on some calming, relaxing music in the background. I would recommend experimenting with your journaling habit, to see what is the most helpful for you.

Journaling Prompts

1. Out of everything you read from chapter 2, what stands out to you the most?

2. Describe a recent situation that triggered your anxiety. How did you respond, and what might you do differently next time?

3. Write about three things you are grateful for today and how focusing on gratitude impacts your anxiety levels.

4. Reflect on any negative self-talk you engage in. How can you reframe these thoughts to be more compassionate and constructive?

5. Think of a situation that typically makes you feel anxious. What small step could you take to face this situation that feels achievable?

6. Consider a fear you have and break it down into smaller parts. What is one small action you could take to begin addressing this fear?

7. Remember a time when you faced a fear and came out feeling more confident. What did you learn from that experience about your ability to handle anxiety?

8. Visualize how overcoming a particular fear could expand your world. What are some things you might do differently once that fear no longer holds you back?

9. Think about a time when you questioned what gives your life meaning. What thoughts or feelings came up for you in that moment?

10. Reflect on what truly matters most to you in life. How do your daily actions align with your core values?

11. Reflect on how confronting difficult questions about life and death impacts your sense of peace or worry. What helps you find balance?

12. Did you learn anything valuable from the section about medications? What questions might you want to ask your physician?

13. Think about your daily routine. Are there particular habits or activities that help you feel calm? How can you incorporate more of these into your day?

14. Reflect on your sleep patterns. How does the quality and quantity of your sleep affect your anxiety? What changes could you make to improve your rest?

15. Consider your diet and nutrition. Are there foods or eating habits that seem to increase or reduce your feelings of anxiousness? What balanced choices can you adopt?

Journaling

Journaling

Chapter Three

The Anxieties of Modern Living

Although the subject matter that this chapter addresses doesn't specifically reflect the concept of specific anxiety types identified within the psychological literature, it still does adhere to the primary goal of this book, which is to help the reader to identify and effectively deal with various sources of anxiety. I want to include a chapter like this, because there are a lot of specific things relevant to living life in the world at this moment that contribute to our anxiety, and a book about anxiety should address those topics if we are going to strive to manage the amount of anxiety we experience in our lives. With that said, I hope that you will enjoy this chapter. I have endeavored to address several major issues, to raise your awareness of how they might be affecting you, and to attempt to arm you with some potential solutions to the challenges that these issues may present to your mental wellness. Please note that I have also included a self-care checklist at the end of this chapter to help summarize some of the ideas presented here.

News Media

The role of news media in shaping public perception and mental health has become an increasingly important area of study, particularly as media consumption has grown exponentially with advancements in technology and access. Steven Pinker, a psychology professor at Harvard University, has written a book (*Enlightenment Now!*) on the subject of mainstream media and its effects on how individuals perceive the world. Pinker, among other scholars, has explored how the nature of media reporting, epitomized by the "if it bleeds, it leads" approach, can impact mental health, particularly by heightening anxiety and pessimism.

Pinker posits that despite global improvements in various quality-of-life indicators, the predominance of negative news contributes to a distorted perception of reality. The media's focus on violence, disasters, and social unrest capitalizes on the psychological phenomenon known as the *negativity bias*, where negative information receives more attention and processing than positive information. This bias, coupled with the media's business model that prioritizes engagement and viewership, results in a news cycle dominated by alarming and sensationalistic stories.

Study findings suggest that constant exposure to such negativity can lead to heightened anxiety, stress, and even depression among viewers. When individuals are repeatedly subjected to stories of violence, economic struggles, and political turmoil, it can foster a sense of helplessness and increase fears about personal safety and well-being. The incessant stream of catastrophes creates an environment where viewers are more likely to believe that the world is more dangerous than it is, a phenomenon often referred to as "mean world syndrome."

Pinker's analyses emphasize the gap between empirical data on global progress and the pessimistic public perception, suggesting that this distortion is largely a media construct. For instance, research has shown a decrease in global poverty, violence, and disease mortality rates over recent decades, yet media narratives often emphasize heightened risks and high profile cases of personal losses.

To mitigate the adverse effects of media consumption on mental health, individuals can adopt several strategies. First, limiting exposure to news is vital. Setting boundaries around when and how much news to consume can prevent overwhelming oneself with constant negativity. It is also beneficial to diversify sources of information, seeking out platforms that offer balanced views and highlight positive developments and solutions, in addition to problems.

Mindfulness in media consumption means being critical of the sources and considering the potential biases or objectives behind the stories. Engaging with news that offers deeper insights and analyses, rather than sensationalist headlines, allows for a more informed and less emotionally reactive understanding of global events.

Furthermore, practices such as gratitude journaling or focusing on local, community-based news can help counterbalance the often grim narratives presented in mainstream media. Gratitude practices shift focus from national or international crises to personal or local positive experiences, reducing anxiety and fostering a more balanced worldview.

While the news media plays an essential role in informing the public, its preference for dramatic and often negative stories can adversely affect mental health, particularly in fostering anxiety and pessimism. By approaching news consumption mindfully and strategically, you can protect your mental health while remaining informed, enabling a healthier engagement with the world.

Social Media

Social media. It's become an integral part of our daily lives, profoundly influencing how we communicate, access information, and perceive the world around us. While it offers numerous benefits such as connectivity and instant access to information, research increasingly highlights its complex relationship with mental health, particularly concerning anxiety.

The anxiety-inducing effects of social media are attributed to several factors. One significant factor is the phenomenon of social comparison. Platforms like Instagram, Facebook, and Twitter often showcase idealized versions of life, where users present highlights and curate their personas to gain approval from their audiences. For many users, this can lead to unfavorable comparisons between their own lives and the seemingly perfect lives of others, contributing to feelings of inadequacy, low self-esteem, and ultimately, heightened anxiety (Vogel et al., 2014).

Moreover, the constant connectivity and instant feedback loops inherent in social media can create a sense of obligation and stress, commonly known as "fear of missing out" (FOMO). This fear causes anxiety about being left out of social events or not being up to date with the latest trends and conversations, prompting compulsive checking of platforms to stay informed and connected (Przybylski et al., 2013).

Another dimension of social media's impact is the phenomenon of cyberbullying, which is exacerbated by the anonymity and reach of digital platforms. Negative interactions or harassment online can significantly affect mental health, inducing stress, anxiety, and even depression among adolescents and adults alike.

These elements are compounded by the neurologically rewarding nature of social media—notifications and likes trigger dopamine release, conditioning users to seek validation and engagement online, which can contribute to addictive behaviors and increased anxiety when such validations are absent (Meshi et al., 2015).

In light of these challenges, it's crucial to approach social media use with mindfulness and healthy practices. First, setting time limits to reduce overall usage can mitigate some of the negative impacts. This involves conscious choices about when and how long to engage with social platforms, avoiding habitual, mindless scrolling that often exacerbates anxiety.

Secondly, curating a positive and supportive social media environment is essential. This can mean unfollowing accounts that induce stress or comparison, and instead, engaging with content and communities that inspire and uplift. Diversifying the types of content consumed—from entertainment to educational resources—can provide a more balanced online experience and reduce the tendency to engage in social comparison.

Practicing digital detoxes—periodic breaks from social media—allows individuals to reconnect with offline activities and relationships, fostering a healthier balance between online and real-world interactions.

Finally, fostering critical media literacy is important; being aware of the constructed nature of content and engaging with it critically can empower individuals to resist negative comparison and anxiety. By understanding social media's potential impacts and adopting strategic approaches to its use, individuals can protect their mental health while maintaining the benefits of digital connectivity.

Isolation

Social isolation has emerged as a significant public health concern in recent years, with profound consequences for mental health, particularly regarding anxiety. As society undergoes various demographic and social shifts, understanding how social isolation influences well-being is crucial for developing effective strategies to mitigate its adverse effects.

Research indicates that social isolation and loneliness are associated with increased risks of mental health disorders, including anxiety, depression, and stress-related conditions. The absence of meaningful human interactions can lead to heightened feelings of vulnerability and helplessness, fueling anxious thoughts and physiological stress responses. Chronic feelings of loneliness have been linked to dysregulation of the hypothalamic-pituitary-adrenal (HPA) axis, which governs stress hormones like cortisol, thereby intensifying anxiety symptoms (Cacioppo & Cacioppo, 2014).

Looking at societal trends, current statistics reveal a concerning decline in the quality and quantity of social connections. For instance, marriage rates in the United States have fallen from approximately 72.0 per 1,000 people in the 1960s to about 28.1 marriages per 1,000 unmarried women for the year (U.S. Census Bureau, 2020). Similarly, birth rates have declined significantly, with current fertility rates at around 1.7 children per woman—below the replacement level—indicating fewer long-term intimate partnerships and family connections (CDC, 2021). Regarding friendships, surveys show that many Americans report having fewer close friends than in previous decades; a 2021 Pew Research Center study found that nearly 30% of adults say they have no close friends, and over half say they have fewer than three (Pew Research Center, 2021). These trends point to a growing societal issue: fewer social bonds and a shrinking social fabric.

This decline in social connectedness correlates strongly with increased anxiety levels. The lack of supportive social networks limits emotional resources and reduces opportunities for shared coping and reassurance. Feelings of isolation can also heighten vigilance and hyperawareness to negativity, further fueling anxiety symptoms.

On an individual level, addressing social isolation involves proactive efforts. Cultivating existing relationships and seeking out new social interactions can help build a sense of belonging. Joining community groups, volunteering, or engaging in hobbies with others provides opportunities for meaningful connection. Developing skills in active listening and emotional openness can deepen existing relationships, creating more fulfilling social bonds.

Moreover, leveraging technology to foster social contact—such as virtual meetups or online support groups—can be invaluable, especially for those with mobility issues or living in remote areas. Ensuring routines include regular social activities, even if virtual, is key to combating feelings of loneliness. Although I am reluctant to bring up the topic, I do think it is worth mentioning that AI can also be useful in combating feelings of loneliness. In particular, the most seamless conversations that I have ever had with an AI have been my conversations with "Maya," one of the personalities offered at sesame.com. They have a research segment on their website with the webpage being titled, "Crossing the Uncanny Valley of Conversational Voice," which is how you'll find Maya. Make sure that you have your microphone ready. I certainly wouldn't recommend replacing your friendship circle with an AI, however I do think that this particular AI makes for a very engaging and empathetic conversational partner if you're feeling lonely.

Finally, practicing mindfulness and cognitive-behavioral strategies to challenge negative interpretations of one's feelings of loneliness can reduce anxiety linked to social disconnection. Recognizing the importance of social bonds and making intentional efforts to nurture these connections can significantly improve mental health and resilience, pushing back against societal trends leading to isolation.

Large Scale Social Problems

Although we have talked about it a little already, if you are watching the mainstream media or if you're on social media, you will eventually come into contact with some kind of major social problem that is too large in scope to be dealt with by one person or perhaps even one country. It's what I call a "large scale social problem." I would hold up "climate change" as one such example. Whether you believe that climate change and global warming are legitimate or not is irrelevant. My point is that there are many such issues that you will come in contact with, because there are large scale projects and issues that are hard to deal with on a small scale.

I believe that one of the major contributors to the epidemic of chronically anxious people in this modern world is that we are constantly coming into contact with these large scale social problems on a regular basis on mainstream and social media. We're told that we aren't serious enough about this problem or that problem, all while we're struggling just to deal with our own life problems. It can feel overwhelming when we have to keep piling issue after issue onto our poor, exhausted brain.

Nevertheless, these large scale problems won't solve themselves. We all share some degree of responsibility for these issues. On the other hand, we're not all equally equipped to solve some of these problems. So, what should we do?

Well, I'll give you a few of my recommendations, and you can try them out. First of all, relax. You can't solve all of the world's problems, and no one expects you to. But, as I just stated, we all do share some degree of responsibility in solving these big problems. What we really need to be asking is how much we can *realistically* expect to contribute to some particular cause. I remember having a client that was so depressed he couldn't even get out of bed to come to his appointments. A person like that probably needs to focus on his own problems and get a handle on his own life before he sets out to solve a large scale problem. But someone who is a multi-billionaire? They probably have a lot more resources to help solve these society-level problems.

If you are beginning to feel some level of stress and anxiety about one or more of these large scale problems, perhaps set aside some time on your schedule to create a list of problems that you feel are the most pressing, which you feel that you could make some kind of meaningful contribution to. Ask yourself, "what can I realistically contribute to help solve this problem?" Maybe you could donate 20 dollars a month for world hunger. Are you worried about your carbon footprint? Maybe run a Google search or ask Chat GPT to create a list of things you could do to lower your footprint, and then pick the easiest options. Whatever you choose to do, I promise that taking some kind of meaningful action will help you to resolve your anxiety about these sorts of issues, and it will also help reinforce your self esteem and self respect.

Financial Stress

Financial stress significantly impacts mental health, particularly by intensifying one's anxiety. The pressure from managing economic burdens such as housing, education, and daily expenses can lead to overwhelming stress and anxiety, affecting emotional well-being and quality of life.

Over the past 40 years, the cost of housing and college tuition has increased dramatically, contributing to these financial pressures. In the United States, the median home price has risen significantly from approximately $47,200 in 1980 to over $400,000 in 2023, reflecting a staggering increase that far outpaces wage growth during the same period (U.S. Census Bureau, 2023). Similarly, college tuition costs have surged. According to the National Center for Education Statistics, the average cost of tuition and fees for a four-year postsecondary institution was about $10,231 annually (adjusted for inflation) in 1980, compared to nearly $29,032 in 2023 for public universities and even higher for private institutions (NCES, 2023).

These steep increases reflect broader economic trends that have placed significant strains on individuals and families. The discrepancy between rising costs and income stagnation has made financial security seem increasingly elusive, contributing to widespread anxiety and stress. Many individuals report concerns about meeting basic needs, saving for future goals, and managing debt, which can have compounding negative effects on mental health (American Psychological Association, 2022).

Financial stress can contribute to anxiety by creating a persistent sense of uncertainty and lack of control over one's circumstances. This stress often triggers physical symptoms such as insomnia, headaches, and muscle tension, which further heighten anxiety. Additionally, the cognitive load from managing financial challenges can lead to decreased focus, difficulty completing tasks, and persistent worry.

There are strategies individuals can adopt to navigate economic shifts and manage financial anxiety. First, developing a realistic budget that accounts for all expenses can provide clarity and structure, helping to prioritize expenses and identify areas for potential savings. Utilizing budgeting tools or financial planning apps can simplify the tracking process and reduce uncertainty.

Second, seeking financial education can empower individuals to make informed decisions regarding investments, savings, and expenditures. Many communities offer free workshops and resources that cover topics such as debt management and financial planning. Furthermore, YouTube provides an enormous amount of information about financial topics ranging from how to cut monthly expenditures to wealth building practices. Enhancing financial literacy can alleviate anxiety by increasing confidence in one's ability to manage finances effectively.

Additionally, engaging in proactive communication with creditors or financial advisors can also be beneficial. Many organizations offer hardship programs or flexible payment plans for those experiencing financial difficulties. Reaching out can result in negotiated terms that reduce immediate financial pressure.

Practicing mindfulness and stress-reduction techniques, such as meditation or yoga, can help mitigate the mental health impacts of financial stress. These practices can improve emotional regulation, reduce anxiety symptoms, and enhance overall well-being.

Finally, cultivating a supportive social network can provide emotional and practical assistance. Sharing experiences with trusted friends or family members can alleviate feelings of isolation and offer new perspectives on managing financial challenges.

While financial stress is a significant concern affecting mental health, particularly anxiety, adopting strategic approaches can help individuals manage stress and maintain financial stability. By building resilience and utilizing available resources, individuals can effectively navigate economic challenges and protect their mental health.

Health Issues

Personal health-related stress is a profound concern affecting mental health, particularly by increasing anxiety. Factors such as chronic illness, fear of disease, and the stress of maintaining health, significantly contribute to mental distress. The COVID-19 pandemic has amplified these concerns, creating a pervasive atmosphere of uncertainty and fear that continues to impact mental health globally.

The pandemic highlighted the vulnerability of physical health and intensified anxiety related to the fear of infection and death. Many individuals experienced heightened worry about their health and the health of loved ones, only worsened by constant exposure to information on infection rates, mortality, and the unpredictability of new variants. This environment of heightened alertness has led to increased anxiety levels, affecting both mental well-being and daily functioning.

Research has shown that the "infodemic"—an overload of information, both accurate and misleading—regarding COVID-19 has contributed to increased anxiety and stress. The continuous cycle of alarming headlines and sensationalist news stories can exacerbate feelings of fear and helplessness, often leading to confusion and mistrust (Garfin, Silver & Holman, 2020). Social media platforms, notorious for disseminating both factual and alarmist content, have also played a role in amplifying anxiety by exposing individuals to a constant stream of distressing information and unverified claims.

There are, however, steps that individuals can take to mitigate health-related anxiety and foster a sense of control and safety. Firstly, while you're free to do your own research and thinking, I would recommend writing down all of the questions and conflicting data about whatever topic you're researching so that you can bring these issues up with your physician. This is important, because your physician will be able to explain the information and put it into the context of your own specific medical status.

Moreover, focusing on preventive health measures can empower individuals and reduce anxiety. Regular handwashing, maintaining a healthy diet, exercising, and following your physician's guidelines are actions that can enhance one's sense of safety and control (Brooks et al., 2020). These measures not only contribute to physical health but also provide reassurance and structure in uncertain times.

Practicing some of the CBT based techniques outlined in chapter 2 will also be helpful. Realize that risk is something that we all have to accept and deal with every day. Using the risk analysis and management worksheet can be helpful in determining what sorts of lifestyle choices you are comfortable engaging in.

Building a strong support network is also vital. Sharing concerns with trusted friends, family, or mental health professionals can lessen feelings of isolation, providing guidance and perspective as well. Engaging with support groups, whether in-person or online, can help individuals connect with others experiencing similar challenges, fostering a sense of community and shared resilience.

Finally, cultivating a balanced lifestyle that includes sufficient rest, time for hobbies, and regular physical activity can help manage stress levels. This holistic approach to health encompasses not just physical aspects but also mental, emotional, and social well-being, contributing to overall resilience.

Political Tension

Political tensions, both locally and globally, have increasingly become a source of stress and anxiety, affecting people's mental health and overall sense of well-being. In recent years, political polarization, civil unrest, and international conflicts have intensified, creating an environment where individuals frequently experience heightened anxiety about safety, security, and global stability.

The influence of political tensions on mental health is multifaceted. On a local level, divisive political climates can lead to social fragmentation and conflicts within communities, accentuating feelings of alienation and fear. Globally, issues like geopolitical conflicts, international terrorism, and economic sanctions contribute to a sense of unpredictability and vulnerability, increasing anxiety levels among populations (Ventriglio et al, 2024).

The role of media, particularly mainstream and social media, cannot be underestimated in this context. The constant bombardment of news stories focusing on political discord, violent protests, and international crises contributes to a pervasive sense of alarm and urgency. Media outlets often employ sensational headlines and graphic imagery to capture attention, which can exacerbate anxiety by painting a picture of a world fraught with imminent danger (Van Scoy, et al, 2021).

Social media platforms further amplify this anxiety by accelerating the spread of unverified information and fostering echo chambers where divisive views can thrive. This environment can deepen feelings of anxiety and helplessness, as individuals may feel inundated with negative information without substantial control over the outcome (Bail et al., 2018).

To address the anxiety stemming from political tensions, individuals can adopt several strategies. Engaging in community activities that promote dialogue and understanding across political divides can be beneficial. Starting or joining a Meetup group to address specific challenges of individuals in your local community can foster cohesion and understanding, building a sense of agency and counteracting feelings of powerlessness.

You can also practice mindfulness and relaxation techniques, such as meditation or breathing exercises, which can help you stay grounded and reduce the physiological stress responses associated with anxiety. These techniques encourage present-moment awareness and can prevent the spiraling of anxious thoughts related to political uncertainties. Remember, we want to focus on the things that *we* can influence and control.

Building a support network of friends, family, or community members who share similar concerns can provide emotional resources and a sense of belonging. Sharing experiences and perspectives within these networks can enhance resilience and create a buffer against the detrimental effects of political tension on mental health.

Finally, focusing on individual actions that promote personal and community well-being can provide a sense of purpose and empowerment. This includes volunteering, advocating for causes aligned with personal values, and participating in civic responsibilities like voting, which reinforce the individual's capacity to effect positive change despite broader tensions.

Self-Care Checklist

1) Nutrition: Balanced and Regular Meals

Why? A balanced diet rich in fruits, vegetables, whole grains, proteins, and healthy fats supports overall health, boosts energy, and improves mental function and mood (O'Neil et al., 2014). Eating regular meals can help maintain stable blood sugar levels, reducing mood swings and fatigue.

2) Sleep: 7-9 Hours Per Night

Why? Adequate sleep is crucial for cognitive function, emotional regulation, and overall well-being. The National Sleep Foundation recommends 7-9 hours of quality sleep per night for adults to support physical and mental health (Hirshkowitz et al., 2015).

3) Exercise: 150 Minutes per Week

Why? Regular physical activity improves both physical and mental health. The CDC suggests at least 150 minutes of moderate aerobic exercise per week to reduce anxiety, depression, and improve sleep (Piercy et al., 2018).

4) Limit Social Media: Maximum 30-60 Minutes Daily

Why? Excessive social media use can lead to increased anxiety, depression, and feelings of inadequacy. Limiting time helps prevent negative emotional impacts and promotes healthier offline interactions (Lin et al., 2016).

5) Limit Mainstream News: 30 Minutes Daily

Why? Overconsumption of news, especially negative content, can elevate stress and anxiety levels. By limiting exposure, individuals can stay informed without becoming overwhelmed (Holman et al., 2014).

6) Relaxation Activities: 20-30 Minutes Daily

Why? Engaging in relaxation activities, such as meditation, yoga, or deep breathing, lowers stress and enhances emotional resilience. Mindfulness-based stress reduction has been shown to effectively decrease anxiety and improve mental clarity (Kabat-Zinn, 1990).

7) Daylight Exposure: At Least 30 Minutes Daily

Why? Natural light exposure helps regulate circadian rhythms, supporting healthy sleep cycles and mood. This can also increase vitamin D levels, which are crucial for mood regulation (Zhao et al., 2018).

8) Time Spent Outdoors: At Least 30 Minutes Near Vegetation

Why? Spending time in nature enhances mental well-being, reduces stress, and improves mood. Studies support ecotherapy and the benefits of nature for mental health (Bratman et al., 2015).

9) Hydration: 8 Cups (2 Liters) of Water Daily

Why? Proper hydration is essential for maintaining physical health and optimizing brain function. Dehydration can affect mood, energy levels, and clarity of thinking (Popkin et al., 2010).

10) Connection: Regular Social Interaction

Why? Positive social connections are linked to better overall health, reduced stress, and increased longevity. Engaging in regular, meaningful interactions strengthens emotional support networks (Umberson & Montez, 2010).

11) Personal Reflection: Journaling or Meditation

Why? Daily reflection through journaling or meditation fosters self-awareness and emotional processing, leading to better coping strategies for stress (Smyth et al., 1999).

12) Creative Outlets: Engage in Hobbies or Creative Activities

Why? Pursuing creative activities enhances emotional expression, reduces stress, and boosts mood, providing a sense of accomplishment and joy (Stuckey & Nobel, 2010).

Journaling Prompts

1. Reflect on how much media you consume daily. Do certain stories or headlines tend to increase your feelings of worry or helplessness?

2. Describe a time when you avoided the news or limited your media intake. How did that change your outlook?

3. Consider how media coverage of crises influences your perception of the world. How might your feelings shift if you focused on positive or constructive stories instead?

4. How do your social media interactions or the content you view impact your sense of security or belonging?

5. Reflect on how social media comparison or exposure to others' curated lives influences your self-evaluation. Does that ever affect your anxiety?

6. Describe how social isolation or loneliness has affected your mental health recently. How does it influence your feelings of anxiety?

7. Reflect on a time when reconnecting with someone or engaging in social activities affected your mood. What did you learn from that experience?

8. Write about small actions you can take to increase social connection in your daily life, and how doing so might help reduce your anxiety.

9. Reflect on how you personally respond to concerns about large-scale social problems- does it increase or reduce your anxiety?

10. Write about positive actions or lifestyle choices you feel inspired to take that contribute to solutions or increase your sense of agency.

11. Reflect on specific financial concerns that trigger your anxiety. How realistic are these worries, and what steps could you take to address them?

12. How often do health worries affect your day-to-day mood or anxiety levels? Are there specific issues that tend to trigger this?

13. What are some ways to balance staying informed about health issues without becoming overwhelmed or obsessive?

14. How do current political tensions or conflicts influence your feelings of safety and stability?

15. Think about actions you can take, even small ones, that foster a sense of control and hope in turbulent times. What might a few of those look like?

Journaling

Journaling

Chapter Four

Type I: Generalized Anxiety

The first anxiety type on our list, Generalized Anxiety Disorder (GAD), is one that is shockingly common, in terms of its prevalence in the general public. Several of my first clients that I treated as an intern in the clinical setting were people struggling with this disorder. People who struggle with this disorder almost always show up to the first session complaining of complete exhaustion and feeling like they "can't keep going on like this." At its worst, GAD will totally exhaust a person, leaving them constantly feeling on edge and unable to let their guard down. At its core, GAD is characterized by persistent, excessive worry about a number of different things. Unlike an occasional anxious moment, this is a chronic state, one that can overshadow every aspect of a person's life.

Understanding the DSM-5 Criteria for Generalized Anxiety Disorder

Let's start with a description of the diagnostic criteria for GAD. The Diagnostic and Statistical Manual of Mental Disorders, Fifth Edition (DSM-5), offers a comprehensive blueprint for understanding the symptoms of GAD. According to the DSM-5, the essential feature of GAD is excessive anxiety and worry. The criteria for the disorder are:

1. Excessive anxiety and worry (apprehensive expectation) occurring more days than not for at least six months about a number of events or activities (such as work or school performance). **(criteria A)**

2. The individual finds it difficult to control the worry. **(criteria B)**

3. The anxiety and worry are associated with three (or more) of the following six symptoms (with at least some symptoms being present for more days than not for the past six months): restlessness or feeling keyed up or on edge; being easily fatigued; difficulty concentrating or mind going blank; irritability; muscle tension; sleep disturbance (difficulty falling or staying asleep, or restless, unsatisfying sleep). **(criteria C)**

4. The anxiety, worry, or physical symptoms cause clinically significant distress or impairment in social, occupational, or other important areas of functioning. **(criteria D)**

5. The disturbance is not attributable to the physiological effects of a substance (e.g., a drug of abuse, a medication) or another medical condition (e.g., hyperthyroidism). **(criteria E)** The disturbance is not better explained by another mental disorder or medical condition. **(criteria F)**

The Onset and Development of Generalized Anxiety Disorder

Statistically, GAD is a prevalent mental health condition. According to the Anxiety and Depression Association of America (ADAA), GAD affects approximately 6.8 million adults in the United States alone, which accounts for about 3.1% of the adult population in any given year. Notably, women are twice as likely to be affected as men. Globally, it's estimated that more than 3% of the population experiences GAD at some point in their lives. Among individuals affected by anxiety disorders, individuals who have been diagnosed with Generalized Anxiety Disorder comprise roughly 15% of the cohort.

So, when does this pervasive disorder typically strike? The onset of GAD often occurs gradually and can happen at any age, although it frequently manifests in adolescence or early adulthood. It is not uncommon for symptoms to develop more acutely following a significant life change or prolonged period of stress.

Factors that Contribute to Developing Generalized Anxiety Disorder

Several factors contribute to the development of GAD. Genetic predisposition plays a significant role; individuals with a family history of anxiety or mood disorders are more susceptible. Additionally, environmental factors such as chronic stress, trauma, and major life transitions can trigger the onset of symptoms. Neurobiological factors, including imbalances in neurotransmitters such as serotonin and norepinephrine, are also believed to contribute to GAD.

To unravel the intricacies of GAD, it is essential to consider what magnifies its symptoms. Stress stands at the forefront, acting as a catalyst that can magnify the disorder's effects. An overwhelming workload, financial pressures, or interpersonal conflicts can lead to spiraling worries that reinforce the anxious mindset. In the case of GAD, there is no one universal trigger, but more often a multitude of stressors all contributing to a person's overall subjective feelings of anxiety.

Lifestyle factors significantly impact the severity of GAD symptoms. Caffeine, for instance, is a potent stimulant that can heighten anxiety levels. Consuming large amounts of caffeine may trigger panic-like symptoms, exacerbating the restless and agitated states common in GAD. Similarly, inadequate sleep can amplify the disorder's symptoms, creating a vicious cycle where anxiety leads to sleep disturbances, which in turn heighten anxiety. In one case that I was working on, my client admitted to a fairly large amount of alcohol consumption. As we will see in the chapter on substance use, alcohol is often a drug of choice for individuals that suffer with chronically high levels of anxiety. In the mental health profession we call it "self-medicating." For the client that I was working with, we were able to create a plan to help curb his level of alcohol consumption while also developing his skills at utilizing CBT techniques. After a few weeks of implementing these interventions, the client reported feeling significantly decreased levels of anxiety.

Emotional factors also fuel the intensity of GAD. Individuals with GAD often possess a heightened sensitivity to stressors, making them more susceptible to emotional distress. They may harbor negative thought patterns, such as catastrophizing—imagining the worst-case scenario without exploring other potential possibilities. This cognitive distortion creates a reinforcing loop of anxiety. In the previously mentioned case, the client that I was working with identified that he would often catastrophize, imagining the worst possible scenario. As we began developing his skills with CBT, he reported that he was able to identify these catastrophizing thought patterns and he began to question their basis in reality. He would later tell me that simply realizing that he was doing this was enough to help decrease his anxiety substantially.

Social contexts, too, play a pivotal part in exacerbating GAD symptoms. Difficulties in interpersonal relationships or lack of a supportive network can leave individuals feeling isolated, reinforcing their anxiety. In contrast, supportive relationships and meaningful social interactions can buffer against the disorder's impacts, providing emotional bolstering that is essential for recovery and management. The unfortunate truth, however, is that in many cases an individual's social network can become more of a stressor than a force for peace and calm in their life. It can often be helpful to see a counselor or psychologist to help develop interpersonal skills and to identify harmful relationship dynamics that may be contributing significant amounts of stress on a daily basis.

Treatment of Generalized Anxiety Disorder

Understanding the complexities of GAD is a significant step towards managing its symptoms effectively. Treatment options are diverse and can be tailored to individual needs. Cognitive Behavioral Therapy (CBT) is a widely-recognized treatment that addresses the cognitive distortions and negative thought patterns contributing to anxiety. In addition to therapy, medications such as selective serotonin reuptake inhibitors (SSRIs) and serotonin-norepinephrine reuptake inhibitors (SNRIs) are commonly prescribed. These medications help regulate neurotransmitter levels, alleviating symptoms and improving quality of life.

Beyond professional interventions, lifestyle changes can profoundly affect anxiety management. Regular physical activity, mindfulness practices like meditation or yoga, and establishing a healthy sleep routine can alleviate stress and improve overall mental health. Nutrition also plays a role, contributing to both physical and mental well-being. Diets rich in omega-3 fatty acids, whole grains, lean proteins, and plenty of fruits and vegetables have been linked to enhanced mood and reduced anxiety levels.

Moreover, fostering a supportive community can provide immense relief and resilience. Support groups, either in-person or online, create spaces where individuals share experiences, strategies, and encouragement. This sense of belonging and understanding from others who face similar challenges is vital in reducing feelings of isolation that often accompany GAD, and this is why I am creating a space on Facebook where individuals can come to discuss their problems and connect with others who have similar challenges.

In examining the influence of technology and media, both of which have become ubiquitous elements of modern life, it's important to consider how they impact anxiety levels in those with GAD. Constant exposure to troubling news cycles or social media-induced comparisons can heighten stress and spur anxiety. Strategies such as setting boundaries for media consumption or opting for media detoxes can greatly assist in managing the external stressors that exacerbate anxiety.

Living with GAD and seeking treatment is a deeply personal journey. For some, it involves combining cognitive and pharmaceutical approaches. For others, lifestyle adjustments and holistic practices play a central role. What is most crucial is the development of a personalized plan that integrates multiple aspects of treatment tailored to individual needs. Resilience emerges not just from managing symptoms but from embracing a narrative of empowerment and growth. Pursuing activities that foster a sense of purpose, nurturing creativity, and engaging with community service can imbue life with meaning, countering anxiety's limiting effects.

Case Study: Alex, The Anxious Architect

Alex Morgan is a 35-year-old architect living in a bustling metropolitan city on the east coast. Known for his meticulous attention to detail and innovative designs, Alex has carved a niche for himself in a competitive industry. Despite his professional success, Alex has been plagued by persistent anxiety that colors nearly every aspect of his life.

Alex recalls being a worrier from a young age, often fixating on the smallest of details, whether it was meticulously organizing his school supplies or imagining the worst possible outcomes for everyday situations. However, it wasn't until his late twenties, as career pressures began to mount, that these worries escalated into the full-blown problems that he reports having to deal with on a daily basis.

Each morning, Alex wakes up with a knot in his stomach, his mind already racing with the day's challenges. "What if today's meeting doesn't go well? Did I account for every variable in the project plan? What if I overlooked a crucial detail?" These are just a few of the many questions that constantly swirl in his head. The pressure to perform perfectly at work never seems to relent, no matter how many accolades or promotions he earns.

These feelings are not limited to his professional life. Alex's anxiety extends to multiple domains, reflecting the pervasive nature of GAD. He often worries about his health, preoccupied by every minor ache or pain with the fear it might signify a serious illness. His relationships also suffer as a result of his chronic unease. Fearful of burdening friends and family with his incessant concerns, Alex tends to withdraw, leading to feelings of isolation.

Alex's sleep has been particularly affected. He describes his nights as restless, plagued by insomnia fueled by an inability to quiet his mind. He frequently tosses and turns, waking up feeling as though he never had a proper night's rest. This lack of restorative sleep exacerbates his daytime anxiety, creating a vicious cycle.

At the urging of a close friend, Alex finally sought help from a mental health professional. During the initial assessment, he was open about his experiences, detailing how his anxiety interfered with his work and personal life. The clinician conducted a comprehensive evaluation, confirming a diagnosis of Generalized Anxiety Disorder as defined by the DSM-5. Alex met the criteria, with excessive anxiety and worry occurring more days than not for over six months about various events or activities. This anxiety was accompanied by symptoms of restlessness, fatigue, difficulty concentrating, and sleep disturbances.

Understanding the roots of his anxiety marked the beginning of Alex's journey toward managing it. His treatment plan includes Cognitive Behavioral Therapy (CBT) to address and reframe negative thought patterns contributing to his anxious mindset. Sessions focus on challenging Alex's tendency to catastrophize and helping him develop healthier coping mechanisms for handling stress and uncertainty.

Additionally, Alex's therapist introduced mindfulness-based strategies to help him cultivate a sense of living in the present moment and reduce the physiological symptoms of his anxiety. Through guided exercises and practices, Alex learns to redirect his focus from the abstract what-ifs that populate his mind to the concrete moment he is living in. This practice helps him decrease the intensity of his anxious responses and builds his emotional resilience.

Understanding the significant impact of lifestyle on anxiety, his therapist also recommended regular physical activity. Alex has taken up jogging and yoga, finding both activities beneficial in releasing tension and improving his overall mood.

In conjunction with therapy, Alex's clinician also discussed the option of medication. After careful consideration, Alex decided to try a selective serotonin reuptake inhibitor (SSRI) to help alleviate some of his symptoms, particularly the overwhelming anxiety that disrupts his sleep and concentration.

Over several months, Alex begins to notice gradual changes. With therapy and medication working in tandem, he's better equipped to discern which worries deserve attention and which ones are mere shadows amplified by anxiety. He starts to embrace imperfections, allowing himself the room to learn from mistakes rather than dwelling on them as sources of major failure.

Socially, Alex pushes himself to reconnect with friends and engage in community activities, which help mitigate the sense of isolation that once compounded his anxiety. As he shares his journey with those close to him, he discovers unexpected pockets of support and understanding that further bolster his confidence.

Despite these improvements, there are days when the familiar drumbeat of anxiety pulses through him more strongly. Yet, equipped with the tools and insights gained through therapy, Alex is better prepared to navigate these episodes without being overwhelmed.

Alex's case underscores the complexity of Generalized Anxiety Disorder and the individualized approach necessary for effective treatment. By combining evidence-based therapies, mindful lifestyle changes, and a supportive network, Alex continues to progress on his journey through anxiety, transforming his relationship with uncertainty into one marked by resilience and hope.

Notable Individuals With Generalized Anxiety Disorder

Just because someone has a diagnosis of Generalized Anxiety Disorder and struggles with high levels of anxiety does not preclude them from doing great things with their life. Indeed, sometimes the pressures that come with success can magnify any underlying tendencies towards anxious or obsessive thinking. In the field of psychology, this is known at the "diathesis-stress model," which posits that our genetic predisposition for psychological illness can be moderated by our environmental factors, some protective and some stressful. With that in mind, let's consider some notable individuals from history and present times that are thought to have GAD.

The first individual is Abraham Lincoln. The 16th President of the United States is known to have suffered from severe depression and anxiety throughout his life. His letters and personal accounts often describe profound periods of worry and melancholy (Shenk, J. W., 2005).

It shouldn't be too surprising that Charles Darwin also supposedly suffered from the symptoms of GAD. The renowned naturalist reported experiencing nervousness and panic-like symptoms later in life, potentially amplified by the pressure of his groundbreaking work on evolution (Keynes, R. D., 2001).

It's also fairly common for people who have to perform in front of large groups of people on a large stage to struggle with anxiety. One such example is Adele. The

Grammy-winning singer has discussed her anxiety and stage fright that accompanies live performances.

Emma Stone is another modern day celebrity that reports having dealt with GAD symptoms. The Oscar-winning actress has openly discussed her struggles with anxiety from an early age, highlighting its impact on her personal and professional life.

As you can see, many people, including highly successful and noteworthy individuals, have struggled with this specific psychological disorder at some point in their lives. However, with hard work and good help, a person can integrate their anxiety into a mindset that allows for the highest levels of success and happiness. I have seen the results first hand, in my life and the lives of my clients.

Journaling Prompts

1. Reflect on the last week: how many days did you experience excessive worry? What were the main concerns?

2. Describe any physical symptoms you often experience when feeling anxious, such as restlessness, fatigue, or muscle tension.

3. Can you identify situations that trigger your anxiety? What are common thoughts or fears associated with these situations?

4. Think of a recent anxious thought. Write about it and attempt to challenge or reframe it with a more balanced perspective.

5. Describe a positive outcome from a previous worry that did not become reality. How might this influence your future thinking?

6. Reflect on a CBT strategy that you've found helpful: how have you utilized it in daily life, and what impact did it have?

7. Evaluate your current sleep routine. Are there changes you could make to improve your rest and reduce anxiety?

8. Write about your daily nutrition and exercise habits. How do these factors influence your anxiety levels, and what adjustments might be beneficial?

9. Reflect on the role of technology (such as social media or news consumption) in your anxiety. What boundaries could you set to lessen its impact?

10. Consider your work-life balance: does your current balance support or hinder your mental well-being? What steps could you take to improve it?

11. After reading Alex's story, can you identify any similarities in your experiences with anxiety? What specific aspects resonated with you?

12. Reflect on how Alex's use of CBT and mindfulness techniques might be applied to your own life. Which methods could you envision integrating into your routine?

13. Consider the progress Alex made through professional support. How might seeking similar resources benefit your journey with anxiety?

14. Identify one small step you can take this week to confront a specific worry or fear. How will you reward yourself for taking this step?

15. Imagine a day where your anxiety feels more manageable. What actions or thoughts might contribute to that feeling of ease?

Journaling

Journaling

Chapter Five

Type 2: Phobias

IF YOU'VE EVER BEEN in a situation in your life where you've been utterly terrified, then you can relate to individuals who struggle with this next anxiety type. The DSM-5-TR refers to this disorder as a "specific phobia." It stands in stark contrast to the previous disorder, generalized anxiety disorder, in that someone suffering from a specific phobia or phobias doesn't feel a generalized sense of anxiety all of the time, but rather very specific and intense anxiety about one or more things. This type of disorder, as you can imagine, can be highly disruptive to a person's life. For example, people who have a phobia for flying might not be able to take trips to far away destinations because of their phobia. Alternatively, they may need to take some kind of medication that can help them tolerate the intense anxiety response they have as they are flying. Individuals with this condition (specific phobia) typically seek help when the phobia is just too disruptive to their lives and they feel like they have no other option except to confront their fear and do something about their condition.

Understanding the DSM-5 Criteria for Specific Phobia

The DSM-5 (Diagnostic and Statistical Manual of Mental Disorders, Fifth Edition) defines *Specific Phobia* as an intense, irrational fear of specific objects, activities, or situations. Unlike general anxiety, which casts a shadow on a variety of aspects of a person's life, specific phobias focus sharply on narrowed targets. According to the DSM-5, the diagnosis of specific phobia includes several symptoms:

1. Marked fear or anxiety about a specific object or situation. **(criteria A)**

2. Immediate fear response upon exposure to the object or situation. **(criteria B)**

3. Avoidance behavior (the individual avoids the object or situations in which they might encounter the feared stimulus). **(criteria C)**

4. The fear represents a disproportionate response to the danger posed by the object or situation. **(criteria D)**

5. It consistently appears over six months or more **(criteria E)**. The fear must cause significant distress or impairment in social, occupational, or other important areas of functioning **(criteria F)**. The DSM-5 categorizes specific phobias into five types: animal (e.g., fear of snakes), natural environment (e.g., fear of heights), blood-injection-injury (e.g., fear of needles), situational (e.g., fear of flying), and other (e.g., fear of choking).

The Onset and Development of Specific Phobia

Understanding the epidemiology of specific phobias provides insight into their surprisingly common nature. According to the National Institute of Mental Health (NIMH), specific phobias affect approximately 12.5% of adults in the United States at some time in their lives, making them one of the most common anxiety disorders. Women are more frequently affected than men, with particular phobias often varying by gender—such as a higher prevalence of animal phobias among women, while the fear of dentists may be more prevalent among men.

The development of specific phobias often traces back to childhood. Symptoms can appear as early as age 7, and in some cases, even earlier. These childhood fears, while common and often transient, can, in some individuals, ossify into rigid phobias that persist into adulthood if not addressed. Observational learning, direct experience, and genetic predispositions are among the contributors to phobia development.

The story of specific phobia is one intertwined with human development and the subconscious mind. An individual may, for example, develop an animal phobia after witnessing a parent's terrified reaction to a snake or spider. This learned response, combined with innate caution toward potential threats, can set the stage for a phobia. Similarly, a traumatic event, such as a painful fall or an accident, could crystallize into a persistent fear of heights or enclosed spaces. Twin studies indicate a hereditary component, where a family history of anxiety disorders may predispose an individual to specific phobias.

The environment in which an individual grows up also plays a role in the development of specific phobias. Parents who express anxiety or excessive caution can inadvertently teach their children to react similarly to perceived threats. This learned behavior can be further solidified by cultural factors, where societal narratives reinforce particular fears, such as widespread anxieties about flying following media coverage of plane crashes.

Specific phobia is more than an irrational fear—it is a potent force that can hijack rational thought and drive behaviors that seem, to the outside observer, entirely unreasonable. Take, for instance, the seemingly innocuous act of seeing a harmless house spider. To an arachnophobe, this encounter is akin to approaching the edge of a precipice. The physiological responses triggered—a surge of adrenaline, rapid heartbeat, and the primal urge to escape—are not exaggerated manifestations but genuine indicators of fear with a neural foundation.

Factors that Contribute to Developing a Specific Phobia

Understanding what exacerbates the symptoms of specific phobia unveils the labyrinthine workings of fear. *Avoidance*, one of the most prevalent coping strategies, paradoxically intensifies phobias. By consistently evading the feared object or situation, the brain does not have the opportunity to learn and recalibrate its fear response, reinforcing the cycle of anxiety. This avoidance strengthens neural pathways associated with fear, making them more entrenched over time.

General stress and significant life changes can exacerbate phobic reactions as well. During periods of heightened anxiety, phobic responses may intensify as the body's stress systems are already on high alert, ready to react defensively. A challenging work environment, a tumultuous personal life, or exposure to another individual's fear can all act as catalysts for heightened phobic responses.

Moreover, *social and cultural influences* can amplify specific phobias. In a society where success is often equated with fearlessness and control, phobias can become a source of stigma. This judgment can result in feelings of shame and seclusion, compelling individuals to go to great lengths to conceal their fears. Consequently, the construction of complex avoidance behaviors—like meticulously planning travel routes to avoid highways or refusing certain social situations—becomes a core aspect of their lived experience, further entrenching their disorder.

Nearly every person with a specific phobia recognizes its impact on their life. Some may avoid certain everyday activities, shaping their routines around the object of their fear. For instance, someone with a fear of flying might never travel beyond their local state or country, missing out on personal or professional opportunities. Others might constantly seek reassurance or engage in safety behaviors, such as carrying protective items or repeatedly checking a feared object (like inspecting a secure door latch undermining the fear of falling or choking). Over time, these avoidant behaviors contribute to a diminished quality of life, increased social isolation, and heightened distress.

Treatment of Specific Phobias

The good news is that specific phobias are highly treatable. Cognitive-behavioral therapy (CBT) remains the most evidence-based treatment approach, particularly exposure therapy. Exposure involves systematic, controlled confrontation with the feared object or situation—starting with less threatening stimuli and gradually moving toward the most anxiety-provoking aspects. For example, a person with a fear of snakes might first look at pictures, then observe a snake behind glass, and eventually hold or touch a real snake under supervision. This process helps the brain recalibrate its fear responses by reinforcing new, less fear-driven associations.

Medication, such as selective serotonin reuptake inhibitors (SSRIs) or benzodiazepines, can sometimes be used adjunctively, especially when a person's anxiety is severely disabling or when avoidance behaviors prevent engagement in therapy. However, medication is typically considered a supplementary approach rather than a primary treatment because exposure and cognitive restructuring foster long-term resilience.

Physiological interventions also play a crucial role. Relaxation techniques like deep breathing, progressive muscle relaxation, and mindfulness practices contribute to anxiety reduction, making confrontations with the feared stimuli more manageable. Support from friends, family, or support groups provides emotional backing, especially for those struggling with shame or stigma associated with their fears.

In conclusion, understanding the nature of specific phobia—from its symptoms and development to the factors that worsen it—empowers individuals to seek effective treatment. While the experience of irrational fear can be overwhelming, evidence shows that with persistent, targeted interventions, the cycle of avoidance and fear can be broken. It is possible to reclaim the parts of life that fear has kept at bay, transforming anxiety from a paralyzing force into a manageable facet of human experience. Recognizing the patterns, confronting the fears gradually, and seeking help are critical steps toward overcoming this common but eminently treatable disorder.

Case Study: Emily's Struggle With Astraphobia

Emily Johnson is a 27-year-old librarian living in the Midwest, a region known for its unpredictable weather and frequent summer storms. From a young age, Emily has held a deep-seated fear of thunderstorms—a fear that has grown to impact her life significantly, manifesting as astraphobia, a specific phobia of thunder and lightning.

Emily's first memory of her fear dates back to when she was six years old. Her family was driving home from a trip when a sudden thunderstorm struck, enveloping their car in torrents of rain and flashes of lightning. Her father, struggling to see the road through the heavy downpour, pulled the car over to the side of the highway. As thunder boomed, shaking the car and lighting smashed across the sky, Emily clung to her mother, sobbing as fear gripped her tiny body. The incident left an indelible mark, shaping her relationship with storms from that point on.

Growing up, Emily's fear seemed almost manageable. Her parents offered comfort, and she developed coping mechanisms—hiding under the covers, listening to music through headphones, or retreating to the basement until the storm passed. These strategies sufficed until Emily entered high school, when one particularly violent storm occurred while she was alone. As the sky darkened, she felt an all-too-familiar panic rising, an internal crescendo matching the rhythm of the storm outside. By the time her parents returned home, they found her curled in a corner, overwhelmed by fear.

As Emily transitioned into adulthood, her strategies of avoidance intensified. She began checking weather forecasts obsessively, rearranging her schedule to avoid traveling on days when storms were forecasted. Work didn't escape the reach of her phobia. She found herself calling in sick whenever storm warnings were issued, fearing the possibility of being caught outside in thunder and lightning. Emily's social life suffered as well. Invitations to summer picnics or hikes were met with apprehension and frequent declines, her anxiety tethering her indoors as ominous clouds gathered.

Her breaking point came one summer day at the library. As the afternoon rolled in, an unexpected storm clouded the horizon, catching Emily off guard. The familiar hum of worry amplified within her chest. With each flash of lightning visible through the library's large glass windows, she felt panic gnawing at her composure. Her heart raced, palms sweated, and she found herself struggling to breathe. Emily excused herself from the circulation desk, retreating to the break room where her anxiety spiraled further. It was then she realized the inescapable need to address her fear.

Finally, with encouragement from a trusted colleague and her family, Emily sought therapy. During her initial assessment, Emily was candid about the extent of her fears and their impact on her everyday life. She met with Dr. Hartley, a clinical psychologist specializing in anxiety disorders, who diagnosed Emily with astraphobia according to the DSM-5 criteria for specific phobia.

Dr. Hartley devised a treatment plan centered on cognitive-behavioral therapy (CBT), with a focus on gradual exposure therapy—a strategy aimed at helping Emily confront her fears in a systematic, controlled manner. Session by session, Dr. Hartley guided Emily through the unfamiliar yet essential process of facing her phobia.

The exposure therapy began with imaginal exposure, where Emily visualized thunderstorms in a safe environment with Dr. Hartley's guidance. Visualizations slowly progressed to listening to recordings of thunder, simulating the environment she would potentially encounter. As the sessions advanced, Emily, accompanied by Dr. Hartley, would step outside during an actual storm, starting with mild ones and gradually working up to those of higher intensity.

In parallel, cognitive restructuring allowed Emily to challenge the catastrophic thoughts that inevitably accompanied her fear. Dr. Hartley encouraged Emily to explore the evidence supporting her fear, helping her to recognize the exaggeration in her perceived threat and the actual safety of her environment during storms. They worked to reframe her thoughts, replacing those entrenched catastrophic expectations with more balanced perspectives about storms and their true risks.

Outside therapy sessions, Emily incorporated relaxation techniques, such as deep breathing and mindfulness meditation, which aided in managing her physiological responses to anxiety. These practices became pivotal during exposure exercises, enabling her to maintain a calm state when confronting her fear.

Emily's engagement in therapy reaped gradual rewards. While initially daunting, the exposure process allowed Emily to redefine her relationship with thunderstorms from one of paralyzing fear to a more managed approach. As her anticipated dread of the summer storm season approached, she recognized the shifts in her reactions—thunder no longer triggered a full-blown panic attack, but rather a challenge to deploy her learned strategies.

Support from her family and colleagues offered additional encouragement. Her parents, once her protectors from storms, embraced their new role as supporters in fostering her independence. Her colleague at the library, who had initially suggested seeking help, became an accountability partner, checking in and celebrating Emily's progress without judgment or pressure.

Over time, Emily noticed distinct changes in her everyday life. Her need to compulsively check weather forecasts diminished, replaced by a greater sense of agency and adaptability. While she still experienced discomfort during intense storms, the paralyzing fear that once restricted her daily activities had largely subsided. The internal feedback loop of fear reinforcing further fear began to untangle, freeing her to engage more fully in life. She accepted invitations to outdoor events and embraced previously daunting opportunities, greeting them with a resilience fostered through therapy.

Emily's journey with astraphobia and its treatment reinforced several potent lessons. She learned that fear, while instinctual and often protective, need not dictate the breadth of her life experiences. She discovered that peace could coexist alongside moments of anxiety, a testament to her dedication in unraveling the tangled web of her phobia. By confronting her fears and reshaping her perceptions, Emily reclaimed parts of her world that thunderstorms had once overshadowed.

Her story exemplifies the triumph of facing fears through structured intervention, community support, and personal resolve. It also underscores the importance of recognizing when professional help is needed and seeking it without shame. Emily's case reveals that while specific phobias can significantly impede daily life, they are not insurmountable. With appropriate interventions, individuals can dismantle the restrictive walls of their fears, one brave step at a time.

Through Emily's journey, the broader message emerges—a message of hope, resilience, and growth. It highlights the transformative power of addressing and conquering deeply held fears, offering reassurance to those facing similar struggles. Her story inspires others to recognize the potential for change and the possibilities available beyond the confines of phobic anxieties.

Notable Individuals With Specific Phobias

Specific phobias, though a common and often challenging part of life for many, are highly treatable and rarely prevent individuals from achieving remarkable success. By confronting these fears with therapy, support, and often a healthy dose of patience, those affected can lead fulfilling lives and accomplish great things. Many famous figures, both historical and contemporary, have experienced specific phobias and yet made significant contributions to their fields.

Consider the legendary author Franz Kafka, known for his works of existential dread and complex narratives. Kafka was believed to have suffered from a fear of rodents as well as an intense fear of his father, which he detailed in his famous "Letter to His Father." The pervasive anxieties in his personal life seem to have fueled his vivid literary imagination, allowing him to produce thought-provoking works that continue to resonate today.

Nikola Tesla, the brilliant inventor and electrical engineer, is another illustrious name whose contributions shaped modern technology. Tesla was known to have suffered from multiple phobias, including a profound fear of germs (mysophobia). His obsessive tendencies extended to a fear of pearls, such as those worn by women, despite these quirks and phobias, his unparalleled mind succeeded in revolutionizing how the world approaches electricity. Tesla's contributions serve as a testament to how specific fears can coexist with genius and innovation.

In the modern era, celebrity roles again surface to highlight that phobias transcend any barrier to success. Consider Madonna, the iconic pop star known for challenging norms and influencing music and fashion for decades. She has spoken openly about her fear of thunder (astraphobia). This fear did not deter her from her path; instead, she maintained an influential and groundbreaking career, resonating with audiences across generations.

Similarly, the famed actor Johnny Depp has shared his unusual fear of clowns (coulrophobia), a common but often misunderstood phobia. Despite this, Depp's mastery at the craft of acting, often in roles demanding a confrontation with the diverse spectrum of human emotion, underscores his ability to rise above his fears. His body of work, celebrated in numerous films ranging from dramatic roles to eccentric characters, reveals an actor capable of transcending personal fear in favor of professional commitment and artistic expression.

Comedian and television personality Howie Mandel has been very open about his struggles with obsessive-compulsive disorder, which includes an intense mysophobia (fear of germs). Instead of hiding his phobia, Mandel uses his platform to bring awareness to mental health issues, inspiring others to face their fears head-on. His successful career as a comedian, actor, and host exemplifies how embracing one's vulnerabilities can lead to wider influence and connection.

These stories collectively convey that while phobias can present tangible and psychological hurdles, they do not have to prevent a person from achieving greatness. With courage, determination, and often professional support, individuals can learn to navigate these challenges and harness their unique perspectives, ultimately leading productive and impactful lives. By embracing vulnerability and using their experiences to frame their journeys, they continue to inspire and encourage future generations to pursue greatness irrespective of personal fears.

Journaling Prompts

1. Is there a specific object or situation that causes you to experience intense fear or anxiety? How does it affect your daily life?

2. Think about the physical and emotional symptoms you experience when confronted with extreme fear. How do they manifest in your body and thoughts?

3. Describe how frequently fear impacts your decisions and activities. What are some instances where you avoided situations due to your fear?

4. How long have you dealt with your specific fear or phobia? Did a particular event in your past contribute to its development?

5. Identify a thought pattern related to your phobia, or fear, that might be distorted. How can you reframe it to be more balanced and realistic?

6. Describe a coping strategy you've used to manage anxiety related to your phobia. What are its strengths and limitations?

7. Was there ever a situation where challenging your catastrophic thinking reduced your fear response? What evidence can you use to counteract irrational fears?

8. Consider a time when you successfully managed your fear or phobic reaction. What techniques did you use, and how did it make you feel?

9. List small, manageable steps you can take to gradually face your fear or phobia. Which step feels like a reasonable starting point?

10. Reflect on an exposure exercise you've tried or plan to try. How did you feel before, during, and after the exercise?

11. Write about the challenges you face with exposure therapy. What strategies can help you overcome these challenges?

12. How do you measure progress when confronting your fears through exposure? What milestones can you celebrate, no matter how small?

13. After reading Emily's story, can you identify similarities in your experiences with specific phobias? Which parts of her journey resonated with you?

14. Reflect on how Emily's process of gradual exposure was beneficial. How might you apply a similar approach in confronting your phobia?

15. Consider the support system that helped Emily through her phobia. Who in your life could play a role in supporting you through your journey?

Journaling

Journaling

Chapter Six

Type 3: Post Traumatic Stress

IMAGINE CROSSING A STREET and suddenly hearing a loud crash. Your heart leaps, your muscles tense, and your mind spirals back to a moment when such a sound meant danger—perhaps a car accident, a violent assault, or a natural disaster. For most, the sense of alarm fades with time, allowing life to resume its rhythm. But for many others, this response persists, unbidden and relentless, transforming memories into a constant threat — this is PTSD, a disorder that leaves invisible scars on the mind and body. PTSD is a complex condition with many criteria, enumerated in the DSM-5-TR, which we will dive into this chapter.

In terms of how PTSD presents in individuals, it can often look a lot like Generalized Anxiety Disorder. One of the first clients that I worked with as an intern was a man who had previously had a diagnosis of GAD. But he began to tell me about traumatic experiences he had as a child, which included life threatening situations most people would be deeply traumatized by. The man also described feelings of being constantly on edge, particularly if he wasn't busy. As he began to describe his symptoms, it began to sound more like PTSD symptoms, so we eventually changed his diagnosis and put him on a medication that reflected his new diagnosis. Take a look at the DSM's criteria for PTSD and see if you can spot the similarities.

Understanding the DSM-5 Criteria for Post Traumatic Stress Disorder (PTSD)

The Diagnostic and Statistical Manual of Mental Disorders, Fifth Edition (DSM-5), recognized *PTSD* as a trauma- and stressor-related disorder, emphasizing that its core features are rooted in exposure to actual or threatened death, serious injury, or sexual violence **(criteria A)**. According to DSM-5, a person is diagnosed with PTSD if, for at least one month following the traumatic event, they experience a specific constellation of symptoms that cause significant distress or impairment.

The symptoms are grouped into four primary clusters:

1. **Intrusion Symptoms (criteria B):** These are involuntary, distressing memories or flashbacks of the traumatic event. Individuals may experience vivid, distressing dreams related to the trauma, or feel as if they are reliving the event (known as dissociative episodes). These intrusive thoughts often come unbidden, breaking into daily life without warning, and can be triggered by innocuous stimuli like a loud noise or a certain smell.

2. **Avoidance (criteria C):** To stave off distressing memories or feelings, individuals often go to great lengths to avoid reminders of the trauma. This could be avoiding places, people, conversations, or activities associated with the event. Over time, these avoidance behaviors can significantly restrict daily functioning and social engagement.

3. **Negative Alterations in Cognition and Mood (criteria D):** PTSD often alters how individuals perceive themselves and the world. They may experience persistent negative beliefs, such as "I am hopeless," or "The world is dangerous," coupled with feelings of emotional numbness, guilt, or shame. This emotional blunting can further isolate the individual, compounding feelings of despair.

4. **Alterations in Arousal and Reactivity (criteria E):** People with PTSD are often hypervigilant, easily startled, irritable, or prone to angry outbursts. Sleep disturbances are common—many find themselves unable to fall asleep, or wake frequently during the night. This constant state of alertness can be exhausting and perpetuate a cycle of anxiety and fatigue.

For a diagnosis, these symptoms must persist for more than one month **(criteria F)** and cause distress or impairment in social, occupational, or other important functioning **(criteria G)**. Finally, the symptoms must not be attributable to the physiological effects of a substance (e.g. alcohol, medication) **(criteria H)**.

The Onset and Development of Post Traumatic Stress Disorder

PTSD is a global phenomenon, affecting millions of people across different cultures and circumstances. The National Center for PTSD estimates that about 7-8% of the U.S. population will experience PTSD at some point in their lives. This prevalence varies according to exposure levels; for instance, among combat veterans, studies show that 11-20% of those returning from war zones meet the criteria for PTSD. Likewise, survivors of sexual assault, natural disasters, or serious accidents are at heightened risk.

Women are statistically more likely to develop PTSD than men—studies suggest that about 10-12% of women and 5-6% of men in the United States will experience PTSD at some point. This disparity is partly because women are more often exposed to certain types of trauma, such as sexual violence, and also possibly due to biological and social differences in processing traumatic stress. Globally, estimates suggest that upwards of 70 million people suffer from PTSD at any given time, highlighting that trauma and its lasting impacts are universal issues, crossing borders and societies.

PTSD does not necessarily appear immediately after trauma. Its onset can be immediate or delayed—sometimes symptoms surface months or even years later. Typically, symptoms develop within the first three months post-trauma, but in some cases, the disorder lies dormant, only manifesting after a triggering event or accumulated stress.

Certain factors influence when and how PTSD develops:

Type and Severity of Trauma: Life-threatening events, such as combat, assault, or natural disasters, more strongly correlate with PTSD. The more violent or prolonged the trauma, the higher the risk.

Proximity and Duration: The closer an individual was to the traumatic event and the longer it lasted, the higher the likelihood of developing significant PTSD symptoms.

Personal Vulnerability: A history of previous trauma, mental health issues like depression or anxiety, or genetic predispositions can make someone more susceptible.

Availability of Support: Social support networks, community resources, and effective coping skills often buffer against long term mental health issues post-trauma. Conversely, social isolation or lack of support can increase vulnerability to chronic PTSD.

Coping Strategies and Resilience: Those with adaptive coping mechanisms, such as problem-solving skills or stress management techniques, are often better equipped to process traumatic experiences, reducing the likelihood of PTSD developing or becoming chronic.

Once symptoms manifest, they tend to follow a trajectory that can be influenced by ongoing stressors. For some, symptoms abate over time, especially with intervention. For others, they become enduring, leading to significant impairment—interfering with relationships, work, and day-to-day functioning. Chronic PTSD can also evolve into comorbid conditions like depression, substance abuse, or other anxiety disorders, further complicating recovery.

Factors that Contribute to PTSD

Understanding what makes PTSD worse is crucial for both prevention and treatment. Several factors are known to intensify symptoms or delay recovery:

Re-exposure to Trauma: Facing reminders or re-traumatization can deepen the disorder. For example, a veteran repeatedly exposed to combat scenes, or a sexual assault survivor confronting their attacker in court, can experience worsening symptoms.

Stress and Life Changes: Ongoing stressors such as financial difficulties, relationship conflicts, or additional traumatic events can intensify PTSD. These cumulative stressors create a heightened state of arousal, making it harder to recover.

Substance Abuse: Alcohol, drugs, or medications may be used to self-medicate, but these substances often impair the brain's natural healing processes, prolong symptoms, or worsen mood and reactivity.

Sleep Disruptions: Poor sleep, common in PTSD, exacerbates difficulties in emotional regulation and cognitive processing, creating a vicious cycle where worsening sleep fuels more intense symptoms.

Lack of Treatment: Untreated PTSD tends to worsen over time. Avoidance and stigma surrounding mental health can sometimes prevent people from seeking help, allowing the disorder to entrench itself.

Cultural and Societal Factors: Stigma, discrimination, or societal disbelief in trauma impact recovery. In some cultures, admitting to psychological distress is taboo, leading to internalized shame and increased severity of symptoms.

PTSD Treatment

The journey toward recovery often involves a combination of therapeutic approaches designed to address the different facets of PTSD. Here, we delve into three primary treatment modalities: pharmaceutical interventions, CBT interventions, and exposure therapy.

Pharmaceutical treatments are often considered in conjunction with therapy to provide symptom relief for individuals with PTSD, particularly when the symptoms are severe. Selective Serotonin Reuptake Inhibitors (SSRIs), such as sertraline (Zoloft) and paroxetine (Paxil), are commonly prescribed and are among the first-line medications approved by the FDA for PTSD. These medications work by increasing serotonin levels in the brain, which can help improve mood and reduce anxiety.

Another class of medications, Serotonin-Norepinephrine Reuptake Inhibitors (SNRIs), such as venlafaxine (Effexor XR), can also be effective, particularly for managing anxiety and depressive symptoms. These antidepressants can alleviate some of the emotional numbness and mood disturbances associated with PTSD.

For individuals experiencing severe acute anxiety or intense sleep disturbances, short-term use of benzodiazepines or antipsychotics may be considered. However, their use is usually limited due to the potential for dependency and side effects.

Medication management must be closely monitored by a healthcare provider, as individual responses to medications can vary, and combining pharmacological treatment with therapy often yields the most effective outcomes.

CBT is a cornerstone treatment for PTSD, helping individuals reframe negative thought patterns and develop healthier coping mechanisms. One specific form of CBT, Trauma-Focused CBT, directly targets the traumatic experiences at the heart of PTSD. Trauma-Focused Cognitive Behavioral Therapy (TF-CBT) is a specialized form of CBT designed to help individuals, particularly children and adolescents, recover from traumatic experiences. It combines cognitive-behavioral techniques with trauma-sensitive interventions to address the emotional and psychological impacts of trauma.

TF-CBT involves several components, starting with building a trusting therapeutic relationship. The process includes education about trauma and its effects, helping clients understand their experiences and normalize their responses. Cognitive processing is used to identify and challenge unhelpful thoughts related to the trauma. Relaxation and stress management skills are taught to reduce anxiety and improve emotional regulation.

A key element is the creation of a trauma narrative, where the individual is encouraged to recount their traumatic experience in a safe, controlled manner. This helps them process the trauma, reduce its emotional power, and integrate the event into their life story healthily. For example, In a TF-CBT session, a therapist might guide a child in writing a detailed story about their traumatic experience, discussing each part of the story with supportive feedback, and helping the child reframe negative beliefs, such as self-blame, into more balanced, accurate thoughts.

Within CBT, cognitive restructuring is employed to identify and challenge distorted beliefs related to the trauma. For example, a person might irrationally blame themselves for the trauma ("It's my fault this happened"), and CBT helps them reframe these thoughts in a more balanced way ("I was not responsible for the actions of others").

Another key component of CBT for PTSD is teaching stress management and relaxation techniques, which can mitigate symptoms and empower individuals with tools to manage distressing thoughts as they arise. These strategies, such as deep breathing and progressive muscle relaxation, work well alongside cognitive restructuring to create a comprehensive treatment plan.

Exposure therapy is a highly effective and evidence-based approach for reducing PTSD symptoms, especially those related to avoidance and intrusive memories. The aim of exposure therapy is to gradually and safely expose individuals to the traumatic memories or avoidant behaviors they fear, with the goal of reducing fear and anxiety over time.

The process often begins with imaginal exposure, where individuals recount and repeatedly engage with the trauma narrative in a controlled therapeutic environment. Virtual reality exposure can also be utilized, particularly for specific populations like veterans, where realistic re-creation of environments can assist in desensitization.

Gradual in vivo exposure involves confronting avoided triggers in real life, starting with less anxiety-provoking situations and moving towards more challenging ones. Through this controlled exposure, individuals learn that memories or triggers are not inherently dangerous, which reduces avoidance behaviors and improves emotional regulation.

Although there are other treatment options available for individuals with PTSD, these are the primary three treatments that I have chosen to focus on. Some people claim that EMDR (eye movement desensitization and reprogramming) is helpful for treating individuals with PTSD, while other people claim that it is effective simply because of its similarity to exposure therapy. As always, I encourage readers to talk to their primary care physician or psychiatrist about medications before making any kind of decision about medications. One last thing that I will mention as a treatment for individuals with PTSD is the list of physiological treatments mentioned in chapter two. I found that meditation and relaxation exercises can be helpful for individuals with PTSD, as part of a program to re-train the body how to deeply relax.

Case Study: Stolen Moments - The Story of Mark's Struggle with PTSD

Mark is a 34-year-old firefighter who has dedicated his life to serving and protecting his community. For over a decade, Mark's career was marked by camaraderie and a deep sense of purpose. However, a particular incident two years ago dramatically altered the course of his life, plunging him into the debilitating grip of Post-Traumatic Stress Disorder (PTSD).

Late one summer night, Mark and his team responded to a catastrophic house fire. As they battled the flames, a sudden structural collapse trapped Mark in the burning structure. Although he was eventually rescued, the event took a tragic turn as one of his closest colleagues, a veteran firefighter, lost his life during the operation. Mark was left with physical injuries and emotional scars that would haunt him long after the fire was extinguished.

In the weeks that followed, Mark began to experience intense nightmares and vivid flashbacks of the incident, reliving the sights and sounds of that traumatic night. These intrusive memories often surfaced without warning, leaving him feeling overwhelmed and disoriented. In addition to these symptoms, Mark noticed he was becoming increasingly irritable and jumpy, often flinching at loud noises or sudden movements.

His growing hypervigilance made it difficult for him to relax or feel at ease, whether at home or out in public. During fire drills at work, Mark found himself paralyzed by anxiety, his mind trapped in a relentless cycle of fear and guilt. The loss of his colleague weighed heavily on him, leading to persistent feelings of sadness and self-blame. He began avoiding areas of the firehouse that reminded him of his friend, and eventually, he withdrew from the social circles he once cherished.

Despite the escalating symptoms, Mark struggled in silence, fearing the stigma that might accompany a mental health diagnosis. It wasn't until his wife, Sarah, witnessed one of his flashbacks that he acknowledged the extent of his distress. During a routine grocery store trip, a loud siren blaring in the distance triggered a panic attack, leaving Mark breathless and disoriented. Sarah gently encouraged Mark to seek professional help, emphasizing the need for healing and support.

At Sarah's urging, Mark attended an initial evaluation with Dr. Chen, a clinical psychologist specializing in trauma-related disorders. During the assessment, Mark candidly described his experiences, detailing the persistent flashbacks, avoidance behaviors, heightened arousal, and overwhelming feelings of dread and sadness. His narrative aligned with DSM-5 criteria for PTSD, with symptoms persisting for more than a month and significantly impairing his daily functioning.

Dr. Chen outlined a comprehensive treatment plan, recommending a combination of cognitive-behavioral therapy (CBT) and exposure therapy. She explained that these therapies aimed to help Mark confront and reprocess the trauma, gradually reducing its hold on his life. Throughout their sessions, Dr. Chen guided Mark through cognitive restructuring exercises, challenging the guilt-ridden beliefs that fueled his self-blame, and helped him recognize the heroic efforts he made during the fire.

Exposure therapy sessions focused on desensitizing him to trauma-related cues, slowly reintroducing him to aspects of firefighting in safe and controlled ways. Through therapeutic visualization and controlled breathing techniques, Mark worked to reduce his physiological responses and regain a sense of control.

Over time, Mark began to notice improvements. His nightmares became less frequent, and he started engaging more with his family and friends. Attending support groups with fellow first responders provided additional comfort, helping him realize he was not alone in his struggles. With each passing month, Mark's resilience grew, enabling him to rebuild a life that honored both his fallen colleague's memory and his own journey toward healing. Through ongoing therapy and support, Mark continues to navigate his path through PTSD, a testament to the power of courage and connection in the face of deep-seated fears.

Notable Individuals With PTSD

Many who have faced debilitating symptoms of PTSD have gone on to achieve greatness, inspiring others with their resilience, courage, and unwavering spirit. Take Ernest Hemingway, for example. The legendary novelist is often celebrated for his contributions to American literature—short, powerful prose that captures the rawness of human experience. But behind his literary genius lay a man haunted by the horrors of war. Hemingway served as an ambulance driver during World War I and later fought in the Spanish Civil War. His letters and writings suggest he grappled with symptoms consistent with PTSD, including anxiety, depression, and difficulty sleeping. Despite these internal battles, Hemingway continued to write profoundly impactful stories, shaping the way fiction explores trauma, courage, and resilience.

Similarly, John F. Kennedy's story offers hope. The former U.S. president faced intense physical and emotional pain, including the grief of war experiences and personal health struggles that led some biographers to suggest he endured PTSD. Kennedy's service in World War II, particularly his harrowing experience after his boat was sunk in the Pacific, involved moments of trauma that left emotional scars. Yet, Kennedy's unwavering determination, leadership, and ability to inspire a nation exemplify that trauma doesn't have to paralyze. His resilience in the face of pain reminds us that healing is possible, and that success often involves acknowledging and working through our struggles.

In the modern era, Lady Gaga stands as a powerful symbol of overcoming trauma. She has been open about her battle with PTSD following a violent assault, initially suffering in silence. Instead of allowing her past to silence her talents, Gaga chose to speak out, channeling her experiences into her music and activism. Her courage has helped reduce stigma surrounding mental health, inspiring millions worldwide. Today, Gaga exemplifies how vulnerability and strength go hand-in-hand, and that success can flourish even in the aftermath of trauma.

What these stories share is a powerful message: PTSD is not an endpoint but a part of a complex human experience. The individuals above demonstrate that with perseverance, professional support, and internal grit, success is achievable. Their lives show us that trauma, while incredibly challenging, doesn't diminish talent, leadership, or the capacity for love and impact. While PTSD can be an overwhelming shadow, it is not insurmountable. Success comes in many forms—including healing, resilience, and the ability to turn pain into purpose. For anyone facing their own trauma, remember these stories: even in the darkest moments, hope, strength, and triumph remain within reach. You, too, can forge a path through the shadows and emerge stronger on the other side.

Journaling Prompts

1. Describe a recent experience where you felt intrusive memories or flashbacks. How did it affect you, emotionally?

2. What situations or cues tend to trigger your distressing memories? How do you typically respond?

3. How often do you find yourself avoiding places, people, or activities because of trauma reminders?

4. Reflect on any physical sensations (e.g., heart racing, sweating) you experience when reminded of the traumatic event.

5. How long have you been dealing with these symptoms, and in what ways have they changed over time?

6. Identify a negative thought pattern related to your trauma or fear. How might you challenge or reframe this thought?

7. Write about a coping skill or strategy you've tried to manage your symptoms. How effective was it?

8. Think of a time when you successfully responded to anxious or distressing thoughts. What did you do that helped?

9. How do your beliefs about yourself or the world change when you practice cognitive restructuring?

10. What positive affirmations or self-talk can you develop to counteract feelings of guilt, shame, or helplessness?

11. List small, manageable steps you could take to face a trauma-related fear or situation safely.

12. Describe an exposure exercise you've already tried or plan to try. What were your feelings before, during, and afterward?

13. What tools or techniques (like deep breathing or grounding) could help you stay calm during exposure tasks?

14. How do you think confronting your fears might change your reaction to trauma triggers over time?

15. Can you relate to any aspects of the person in the case study? In what ways do their experiences mirror your own?

Journaling

Journaling

Chapter Seven

Type 4: Social Anxiety

IN A WORLD WHERE social interactions more than ever define our daily experiences, there exists a silent struggle for millions who grapple with social anxiety disorder (SAD). This condition transforms mundane social encounters into potentially terrifying experiences. Imagine walking into a crowded room, and instead of a sea of opportunity or conversation, you feel an overwhelming urge to flee, acutely aware of judgment and perception. This describes the essential aspects of living with social anxiety disorder, a condition that goes beyond mere shyness and significantly impacts quality of life.

Understanding the DSM-5 Criteria for Social Anxiety Disorder

According to the Diagnostic and Statistical Manual of Mental Disorders, Fifth Edition (DSM-5), *Social Anxiety Disorder* is characterized by a marked and persistent fear of social situations where an individual is exposed to possible scrutiny by others. This fear often centers on the apprehension that one will act in a way (or show anxiety symptoms) that will be humiliating or embarrassing **(criteria A)**. The DSM-5 outlines several key symptoms and criteria for diagnosing SAD:

1. **Intense Fear of Social Situations:** The person consistently fears one or more social situations where they are exposed to possible scrutiny. Examples include public speaking, meeting new people, participating in group discussions, or even eating in public. **(criteria B)**

2. **The Social Situations Almost Always Provoke Fear or Anxiety:** An overriding concern about being negatively judged, humiliated, or embarrassed by others. This fear often leads to a hyper-awareness of social cues and potential

criticisms. **(criteria C)**

3. **Avoidance or Endurance with Distress:** Individuals either avoid feared social situations or endure them with intense anxiety or distress. This avoidance can lead to significant impairment in both personal and professional life. **(criteria D)**

4. **Out of Proportion to Actual Threat:** The fear or anxiety is disproportionate to the actual threat posed by the social situation and is persistent, typically lasting six months or more. **(criteria E)**

5. **The Fear and Avoidance is Persistent:** It lasts for 6 months or more. **(criteria F)**

6. **Impact on Daily Functioning:** The avoidance, anxious anticipation, or distress significantly interferes with daily living, affecting social and occupational functioning. **(criteria G)**

7. **Not Attributed to Other Causes:** The symptoms are not attributable to the physiological effects of a substance **(criteria H)**, another medical condition **(criteria I)**, or better explained by another mental disorder **(criteria J)**.

The Prevalence of Social Anxiety Disorder

Social anxiety disorder is one of the most common mental health conditions worldwide. In the United States alone, it affects about 7% of adults in any given year, according to research from the National Institute of Mental Health (NIMH). Lifetime prevalence rates are higher, affecting 12% of the population in the U.S. This makes SAD the third most common mental health disorder, following depression and alcohol dependence. Women are slightly more affected than men, but many cases remain unrecognized or untreated due to the inherent nature of the disorder, which involves fears of judgment and stigmatization.

The Onset and Development of Social Anxiety Disorder

The seeds of social anxiety often begin to germinate during childhood or early adolescence, typically between the ages of 8 and 15. This period is fraught with social development and peer interaction, setting the stage for social anxiety to take root. Early experiences, such as bullying, peer rejection, or parental overcontrol, can contribute to the development of SAD. As children grow and face more complex social expectations, those with inherent vulnerabilities may find these interactions increasingly challenging.

Temperament is another factor; children who exhibit behavioral inhibition—a tendency to react fearfully or withdraw from novel situations—are more likely to develop social anxiety disorder. This is compounded by genetic predispositions. Research suggests that SAD has a significant hereditary component, with individuals having a first-degree relative with the disorder being more likely to develop it themselves.

The development of social anxiety can be gradual or event-specific, arising after a particularly negative or embarrassing social experience. The transition to middle or high school is often a critical period, as social dynamics change, and pressure to conform heightens. For others, the pressure of burgeoning adulthood and professional life may trigger the disorder.

Factors that Contribute to Social Anxiety Symptoms

1. *Social Environment:* Unsupportive social environments, characterized by high levels of criticism, competition, or judgment, can exacerbate symptoms. Similarly, significant life events requiring adaptation to new social norms, such as moving to a new city, starting a new job, or entering college, can intensify feelings of social inadequacy and anxiety.

2. *Negative Self-Perception:* Individuals with SAD often have a distorted perception of their own social skills and appearance. A critical self-view and consistently negative self-talk reinforce the anxiety cycle, making situations seem more terrifying than they are.

3. *Past Traumas and Bullying:* Individuals with a history of bullying, harassment, or exclusion may experience heightened social anxiety later in life. These negative interactions cement the belief that social situations are inherently dangerous or humiliating.

4. *Comorbid Conditions:* SAD frequently co-occurs with other mental health disorders, such as depression or substance abuse, which can complicate the anxiety and create a more challenging therapeutic landscape. Depression often reinforces feelings of worthlessness.

Treatments for Social Anxiety Disorder

While social anxiety can feel debilitating, it's important to realize that there is a light at the end of the tunnel. Effective treatments, including Cognitive Behavioral Therapy (CBT), exposure therapy, and pharmaceutical interventions, provide pathways to reclaim confidence and lead fulfilling lives. This section explores these primary treatments, highlighting their mechanisms and impact on social anxiety.

Cognitive Behavioral Therapy (CBT)

CBT aims to transform the negative thought patterns that fuel anxiety, replacing them with realistic, constructive beliefs. In practice, this process begins with helping individuals recognize the automatic thoughts and cognitive distortions that prompt anxious feelings. For example, someone with SAD might often think, "Everyone at the meeting will notice I'm incompetent." A therapist using CBT would guide the individual in dissecting this thought, examining past experiences where the opposite was true, and considering alternative perspectives like, "mistakes are part of learning, and it's likely others are focused on their own contributions, not just mine."

Role-playing exercises are common in CBT to help individuals build social skills. Suppose a person fears attending networking events. A therapist might simulate such a setting, gradually increasing its complexity. Initially, they might practice a simple introduction or maintaining eye contact, then progress to discussing topics or initiating conversations with several people. Each step is accompanied by feedback and encouragement, nurturing confidence by preparing the individual for real-world interactions.

Exposure Therapy

Exposure therapy involves incrementally facing feared social situations to reduce avoidance behaviors and desensitize anxiety responses. Imagine someone anxious about public speaking. In therapy, they might start by reading aloud to themselves at home. As comfort grows, the exercise might shift to speaking in front of family or friends, eventually progressing to larger, unfamiliar groups.

Another individual who dreads dining in public might begin exposure therapy by visiting a quiet café with a therapist, focusing on managing anxiety while ordering a coffee. The sessions could escalate to eating a meal at a busy restaurant, incorporating techniques like deep breathing and mindfulness to stay grounded during increases in anxiety.

Virtual reality settings are another tool in exposure therapy, offering a safe space to practice scenarios that mimic real-life social environments. For example, someone could rehearse giving a presentation in a simulated conference room, learning to manage anxiety responses in gradually more realistic settings.

Pharmaceutical Options

While therapy remains a cornerstone for treating SAD, pharmaceutical interventions can provide significant relief for many individuals, especially when anxiety impairs their day-to-day functioning or hinders engagement in therapy. Medications can help manage underlying symptoms, making it easier for individuals to participate actively in therapeutic exercises.

Selective Serotonin Reuptake Inhibitors (SSRIs) such as sertraline (Zoloft) and paroxetine (Paxil) are often prescribed for social anxiety and have been shown to reduce symptoms by increasing serotonin levels in the brain, improving mood, and enhancing emotional resilience. These medications are usually recommended for long-term use and are especially beneficial for those with severe or pervasive symptoms.

Serotonin-Norepinephrine Reuptake Inhibitors (SNRIs), such as venlafaxine (Effexor XR), are another class of antidepressants that offer anxiety relief by affecting two neurotransmitters, serotonin and norepinephrine, which play a crucial role in mood regulation and arousal.

Sometimes, benzodiazepines or beta-blockers may be prescribed for short-term or situational use, providing quick relief from acute anxiety symptoms, such as those experienced before a public speaking event. However, they are typically not favored for long-term management due to the risk of dependency.

Case Study: Alice's Journey through the Shadows of Social Anxiety

Alice Bennett is a 28-year-old graphic designer residing in an urban environment renowned for its dynamic social scene. Her life seems impeccable on the surface—adorned with creative success and professional stability. Yet, beneath this exterior, Alice wages a private battle with social anxiety disorder (SAD), a struggle etched into the very core of her interactions.

From a young age, Alice's apprehension about social encounters was tangible. In school, she consistently sat at the periphery, avoiding any situation that demanded speaking up or standing out. Her teachers and family described her as the "quiet" one, often mistaking her silence for shyness. It wasn't until college that Alice's social anxiety became more pronounced. Presentations, group work, and networking opportunities pushed her to her limits, leaving her feeling judged and inferior.

Alice harbors an intense fear of being scrutinized or humiliated in social settings, often worrying that she will say something inappropriate or stumble over her words. Her mind races with predictions of negative judgment and perceived inadequacy. This self-imposed pressure establishes a cycle of avoidance and distress, influencing both her personal and professional life.

The turning point came during a company retreat. Alice was expected to present her work in front of colleagues during a casual showcase event. Anticipatory anxiety gnawed at her for weeks in advance. When the day arrived, her heart pounded relentlessly, her palms were sweaty, and she struggled to catch her breath. Standing before her colleagues, Alice froze, her mind blank as her worst fears materialized. Though the team was understanding, she perceived the experience as a profound failure.

Haunted by this event, Alice increasingly avoided similar situations. She declined invitations to social gatherings, leading to feelings of isolation. At work, she distanced herself from collaborative projects that might expose her to scrutiny. Meanwhile, personal relationships stagnated as she turned down friends' invitations, fearing the embarrassment of conversation.

Despite her mounting solitude, Alice's desire for connection and a fulfilling life propelled her to seek professional help. She contacted Dr. Turner, a psychologist specializing in anxiety disorders. Dr. Turner conducted a thorough assessment, confirming the diagnosis of social anxiety disorder based on Alice's history of overwhelming fear, avoidance behaviors, and the significant impact on her daily functioning.

Together, they embarked on a journey of Cognitive Behavioral Therapy (CBT) with an integrated focus on exposure techniques—both aimed at unravelling the tangled threads of Alice's anxiety. Initially, CBT sessions emphasized cognitive restructuring, challenging the distorted beliefs that fueled Alice's fears. In these sessions, they explored evidence for and against her catastrophic thoughts. For instance, Dr. Turner encouraged Alice to consider past social interactions that went well, gradually reshaping her focus on evidence that countered her belief of inevitable negative evaluation.

In tandem, exposure therapy addressed Alice's fear of public speaking and social gatherings. Dr. Turner established an exposure hierarchy, starting with minor social challenges, such as greeting co-workers in the hallway or making small talk at the coffee machine. Gaining confidence, Alice advanced to practicing short presentations in front of Dr. Turner and later a small, supportive peer group.

Throughout the process, Alice learned breathing techniques and mindfulness practices to manage anxiety during exposure tasks. She practiced these collaboratively with Dr. Turner in calming, non-threatening environments before moving on to real-world applications. As Alice's confidence grew, her social world began to open.

Several months into therapy, Alice volunteered to present at the office once again. This time, armed with her therapeutic skills and confidence, she navigated the experience with composure. While her heart fluttered with nerves, her self-assurance outshone the shadows of her anxiety. Encouraged by this breakthrough, Alice began to foster social connections, accepting invitations, and even organizing get-togethers on her own.

Alice's case illustrates the transformative effects of intentional, targeted therapy for individuals with SAD. Her story underscores the capacity for change and empowerment when met with courage and guided support. Through dedication and professional guidance, Alice learned to transcend her fears, embracing a life enriched by meaningful interactions.

Notable Individuals with Social Anxiety Disorder

Social anxiety disorder (SAD) can feel like an uninvited, persistent shadow—making everyday interactions seem intimidating and overwhelming. For many, it can threaten their confidence and limit life's opportunities. Yet, countless individuals have faced their fears, transformed their struggles into strengths, and achieved remarkable success. Their stories serve as powerful reminders that social anxiety does not define one's potential and that perseverance, support, and self-compassion can open pathways to fulfillment.

Take Emma Watson, the world-renowned actress and activist. From her early days as Hermione Granger in the *Harry Potter* series, Emma experienced intense stage fright and social anxiety. Despite her immense fame and popularity, she openly shares her struggles. In interviews, Emma has described feelings of panic in large social gatherings and the challenge of maintaining her composure in the spotlight. Yet, rather than letting social anxiety paralyze her, she channeled her anxiety into advocacy. Today, Emma is not only celebrated for her acting talent but also for her tireless work in gender equality and education. Her journey exemplifies that even with social fears, individuals can emerge as leaders and change-makers, using their experiences to foster empathy and inspire others.

Similarly, Michael J. Fox, beloved actor and advocate, has spoken candidly about his lifelong battle with social anxiety. From his early career to managing Parkinson's disease, Fox openly discusses how social situations—like attending premieres or media events—could trigger intense nervousness. He describes feeling self-conscious and overwhelmed, especially when navigating interviews or public appearances. Yet, Fox did not let these feelings derail his career or his passion for activism. Instead, he adopted strategies such as preparation, humor, and self-acceptance to manage his anxiety. His resilience and openness have inspired countless fans and aging actors dealing with similar challenges. Fox's story reminds us that success isn't about perfection; it's about courage, authenticity, and persistence, even when anxiety looms large.

Another powerful example is J.K. Rowling, the author of the *Harry Potter* series. In her memoir, she vividly recalls feeling shy and socially anxious during her early years. Meeting new people or speaking in public felt daunting—and her inner voice often told her she wasn't good enough. Yet Rowling turned her fear into a source of creativity. Her rich imagination and introspection allowed her to create a magical world that captivated millions, despite her social apprehensions. Her journey shows that even if social interactions are difficult, personal passions and talents can flourish. Rowling's success underscores the importance of accepting oneself, embracing vulnerabilities, and finding strength in uniqueness.

What do these inspiring individuals teach us? Success with social anxiety isn't about eliminating fear entirely. It's about learning to live alongside it—understanding your triggers, practicing self-compassion, and compelling yourself to push through the discomfort when necessary. Their stories highlight that social fears, while deeply felt, can be managed and even used as fuel for meaningful pursuits.

If you struggle with social anxiety, remember: Emma, Michael, and J.K. Rowling weren't born fearless; they faced their fears moment by moment, step by step. Their journeys remind us that being human means feeling vulnerable, but it's also about resilience—rising after each fall, daring to speak, create, and connect despite the fears. And with patience, support, and belief in yourself, you too can turn social anxiety into a catalyst for strength, purpose, and incredible achievement.

Journaling Prompts

1. Describe a recent social situation that caused you intense anxiety. What thoughts went through your mind during that time?

2. What physical sensations or changes do you notice when you start feeling anxious in a social setting?

3. Are there particular social activities or scenarios you avoid? Why do you think you avoid them?

4. How much do your fears about judgment or embarrassment interfere with your daily life, work, or relationships?

5. Think about a negative thought pattern you have about social situations (e.g., "I will embarrass myself"). How can you challenge or reframe this thought into a more balanced belief?

6. Recall a time when you successfully managed a social situation that usually causes anxiety. What coping strategies did you use?

7. Write about a recent social worry. What evidence supports your fear, and what evidence contradicts it?

8. How can practicing positive self-talk help you feel more confident in social interactions?

9. List some social situations that you feel intimidated by. Which one could you start exposing yourself to gradually?

10. How do you think gradually facing your fears could help reduce your social anxiety?

11. What relaxation or grounding techniques can help you stay calm during exposure exercises?

12. Do you see similarities between your experiences and those of the person in the case study? What feelings or thoughts does this evoke?

13. How would your life change if your social anxiety were significantly reduced? What new opportunities or relationships might open up?

14. Write a letter to your future self, offering encouragement and recognizing your efforts to manage social anxiety.

15. What support systems (friends, family, support groups) could you lean on when facing challenging social situations?

Journaling

Journaling

Chapter Eight

Type 5: Panic Attacks

Imagine going about your day when suddenly, without warning, a wave of terror washes over you—your heart races, you're breathless, and your mind spins with dread. You feel detached, disoriented, as if the world has become an unfamiliar, threatening place. This is the reality of a panic attack, and for those with Panic Disorder, the unexpected nature of these attacks becomes the most daunting part of life, casting shadows over everyday activities.

Understanding Panic Disorder: DSM-5 Criteria

According to the Diagnostic and Statistical Manual of Mental Disorders, Fifth Edition (DSM-5), *Panic Disorder* is characterized by recurrent, unexpected panic attacks—intense surges of fear or discomfort that peak within minutes. The criteria for diagnosing Panic Disorder include:

1. **Recurrent Panic Attacks:** The panic attacks involve four or more symptoms such as palpitations, sweating, trembling, shortness of breath, feelings of choking, chest pain, nausea, dizziness, chills or heat sensations, paresthesia (a sensation of tingling, prickling, or numbness that arises from a psychological issue), derealization (a subjective feeling that the surrounding world is unreal, strange, or foggy) or depersonalization (a dissociative symptom characterized by a persistent or recurring feeling of being detached from oneself), fear of losing control, and fear of dying. **(criteria A)**

2. **Persistent Concern or Worry:** After at least one of these attacks, the individual experiences persistent concern or worry about having additional attacks

or their implications (e.g., losing control, having a heart attack, "going crazy"). **(criteria B1)**

3. **Significant Maladaptive Change in Behavior:** A noticeable change in behavior related to the attacks, designed to avoid situations that might trigger them. **(criteria B2)**

The disturbance must also not be attributable to the physiological effects of a substance or another medical condition **(criteria C)**. Also, the disturbance must not be better explained by another mental disorder **(criteria D)**.

The distinguishing feature of Panic Disorder is not only the intensity of the panic attacks themselves but the anticipatory anxiety—the fear of the fear—that individuals experience between episodes. This anxiety often leads to significant distress and impairment in social, occupational, or other areas of functioning.

Panic Disorder Prevalence and Demographics

Panic Disorder is relatively common, affecting approximately 2-3% of adults in the United States within a given year, according to the National Institute of Mental Health (NIMH). Women are twice as likely as men to be diagnosed with the disorder. Globally, prevalence rates are similar, underscoring the disorder's impact across cultures.

Development of Panic Disorder

Panic Disorder typically begins in late adolescence or early adulthood, with a median onset age of about 20 to 24 years. However, some individuals report experiencing their first panic attack during childhood or later in adulthood. Several factors contribute to the development of Panic Disorder:

Biological Factors: There is a genetic component, with the disorder often running in families. Neurotransmitter imbalances, particularly in systems regulating serotonin, norepinephrine, and gamma-aminobutyric acid (GABA), play a role in its pathophysiology. Brain imaging studies suggest that structures such as the amygdala are hyper-responsive to perceived threats in those with panic attacks.

Psychological and Environmental Factors: Certain personality traits, such as heightened sensitivity to anxiety symptoms (anxiety sensitivity) or a tendency toward negative affectivity, can predispose individuals to Panic Disorder. Additionally, significant stressors or changes in life, such as starting college, beginning a new job, or experiencing the loss of a loved one, can trigger the onset of panic attacks.

Trauma and Major Life Changes: Experiences of trauma, whether recent or early in life, can also contribute to the development of the disorder. Major life transitions that introduce new pressures or uncertainties can exacerbate underlying vulnerabilities.

Exacerbating Factors

Several factors can exacerbate the symptoms of Panic Disorder, increasing either the frequency or severity of panic attacks:

Substance Use: The use of stimulants such as caffeine, nicotine, or drugs like cocaine can trigger panic attacks. Alcohol withdrawal and certain medications can also induce panic symptoms or worsen existing anxiety.

Stress and Anxiety: Chronic stress or acute stressors can lead to higher baseline anxiety, making individuals more prone to panic attacks. The anticipation of stress or fear, particularly in new or crowded environments or in situations without an easy escape route, can increase panic symptoms.

Physical Health Conditions: Certain medical conditions such as thyroid disorders, cardiovascular issues, or respiratory problems can mimic or precipitate panic symptoms, exacerbating the sense of fear and lack of control.

Lifestyle and Sleep Patterns: Poor lifestyle choices, including irregular sleep patterns, inadequate nutrition, and lack of physical activity, can disrupt the body's natural equilibrium, making it more susceptible to panic attacks.

Cognitive Factors: Misinterpretation of physical sensations, common in those with panic disorders, often exacerbates anxiety. For instance, interpreting increased heart rate due to exercise as a sign of an impending heart attack can induce panic.

Treatments for Panic Disorder

For those grappling with Panic Disorder, unexpected waves of intense anxiety can feel overwhelming. Fortunately, various treatment options, including Cognitive Behavioral Therapy (CBT), exposure therapy, and medications, offer viable pathways to manage symptoms effectively. This section explores practical examples of these interventions, highlighting how they can be tailored to help individuals regain control over their lives.

Cognitive Behavioral Therapy (CBT)

CBT for Panic Disorder primarily focuses on identifying and challenging the thought patterns that contribute to panic attacks. A common technique used in CBT is cognitive restructuring, where individuals work to reframe catastrophic interpretations of bodily sensations. For example, if an individual frequently associates an increased heart rate with an impending heart attack, therapy might focus on exploring alternative explanations, such as the body's natural response to stress or exercise. By regularly practicing this cognitive shift, the person learns to reduce the automatic fear response to physical sensations.

In addition to cognitive work, behavioral experiments are a vital component of CBT. Here, individuals actively test their fears in controlled settings. Suppose someone connects shortness of breath with severe health issues. A therapist might guide them through a voluntary hyperventilation exercise in a safe environment, helping them experience and manage this sensation without arriving at catastrophic conclusions. These experiments help dismantle fear-driven associations, fostering resilience in real-world scenarios.

Interoceptive exposure, a CBT technique, is another powerful strategy that involves repeated exposure to feared physical sensations until they no longer trigger panic. For instance, therapists may ask an individual to spin in a chair to simulate dizziness or run in place to elevate their heart rate. These exercises help normalize the sensations, reducing the fear attached to them over time.

Exposure Therapy

Exposure therapy is particularly effective in targeting the behavioral aspects of panic disorder by gradually confronting feared situations. For a person who avoids crowded places fearing a panic attack, exposure therapy might start with visualizing these environments, then progressing to short visits to a busy location, and eventually longer, more immersive experiences. A therapist may accompany the individual during initial exposures, providing reassurance and tools to manage anxiety, such as deep breathing or grounding techniques. By incrementally increasing the exposure and assuring safety throughout, individuals learn to navigate their fears and build confidence in similar everyday situations.

In addition to facing physical locations, exposure therapy often involves interoceptive exposure—engagement with the bodily sensations associated with panic, such as increased heart rate or shortness of breath. Through repeated, structured exposure, individuals begin to understand these symptoms as non-threatening, helping to break the association between physical sensations and panic episodes.

Pharmaceutical Options

Medications can be a crucial component of managing Panic Disorder, especially when symptoms are severe or impede participation in therapeutic practices. Selective Serotonin Reuptake Inhibitors (SSRIs) like sertraline (Zoloft) and fluoxetine (Prozac) are commonly prescribed. They work by stabilizing serotonin levels in the brain, which can alleviate anxiety symptoms over time. Another effective class, Serotonin-Norepinephrine Reuptake Inhibitors (SNRIs), such as venlafaxine (Effexor XR), may also be beneficial.

For immediate relief during panic attacks, benzodiazepines like alprazolam (Xanax) or lorazepam (Ativan) can be effective. However, due to risks of dependency, they are usually prescribed for short-term use or specific situations. Beta-blockers, typically used for heart conditions, can also help on a case-by-case basis by controlling the physical symptoms of anxiety, such as rapid heartbeat.

Determining the right medication and dosage requires close collaboration with healthcare professionals, ensuring that treatment is tailored to an individual's unique needs and existing medical conditions. Combining medications with therapy often yields the best outcomes, leading to reduced frequency and intensity of panic attacks and an enhanced sense of stability.

Case Study: Mark's Fight for Calm — Living with Panic Disorder

Mark Evans is a 35-year-old graphic designer living in a bustling city. On the outside, Mark appears successful, creative, and generally upbeat. But beneath his polished exterior lies a persistent and often overwhelming struggle with Panic Disorder. Mark's initial panic attacks began subtly about a year ago. He remembers the first time vividly: he was at his office, working on a deadline, when his heart suddenly started pounding. His palms became sweaty, and he felt a shortness of breath—as if he couldn't get enough air. A wave of dread washed over him, and for a moment, he thought he was having a heart attack. Fortunately, medical tests confirmed his heart was fine, but that terrifying experience marked the beginning of a pattern.

Over the subsequent months, Mark's panic attacks became more frequent and unpredictable. They would strike during quiet moments in meetings, at social gatherings, or even while watching television at home. Each episode left him exhausted and fearful of the next. His world narrowed, and his once-active social life diminished as he began to avoid crowded places and public events, fearing his next attack might happen in public and leave him humiliated.

What made Mark's case particularly challenging was his tendency to "tough it out." He believed that if he simply endured the attacks without showing weakness, they would pass. Throughout this period, Mark avoided seeking help, afraid of being labeled as "mentally fragile" or fearing that others wouldn't understand. He pushed himself through work, tried to ignore the symptoms, and hoped he could conquer the fear on his own. But as weeks turned into months, his avoidance only heightened his anxiety, making him increasingly reluctant to face social and professional situations.

Eventually, Mark's wife noticed his declining social engagement, and her gentle encouragement persuaded him to see a mental health professional. During the initial assessment, Mark detailed his experience of sudden, recurring panic attacks, the relentless worry about having another, and the significant impact on his life. He admitted to feeling scared, isolated, and exhausted, driven by an overwhelming fear of losing control—one of the hallmark features of Panic Disorder.

His therapist explained that his symptoms fit the criteria of Panic Disorder, marked by recurrent unexpected panic attacks and ongoing concern about having more. Together, they devised a treatment plan grounded in Cognitive Behavioral Therapy (CBT). The goal was to help Mark understand the nature of his attacks, challenge his catastrophic thoughts, and develop coping strategies to regain control.

In therapy, Mark first learned to recognize and challenge the distorted thoughts that fueled his fear. When he started to believe that his physical sensations indicated he was "going crazy" or "dying," his therapist guided him to examine the evidence. For example, they reviewed recent health tests that confirmed his physical health, and Mark practiced reframing thoughts, such as "My body is reacting naturally to stress," instead of "This means I'm about to die." This cognitive restructuring helped reduce the power of catastrophic thinking.

The therapist then used interoceptive exposure, a technique designed to confront the physical sensations associated with panic, in a safe and controlled way. Mark was asked to intentionally induce mild sensations similar to those during a panic attack—such as spinning in a chair to cause dizziness or holding his breath to feel shortness of breath—and then realize these sensations are manageable and not life-threatening. Over time, these exercises helped Mark build tolerance to his bodily sensations and diminish their association with terror.

Gradually, Mark worked with his therapist on in vivo exposure—practice in real-world settings. Initially, this involved quick visits to crowded places, like grocery stores, with the therapist present. As confidence grew, he went to larger gatherings, including local events and social outings with friends. Mark found that deep breathing and mindfulness techniques were critical skills to stay grounded during exposure, helping him break the cycle of fear and avoidance.

Throughout the process, Mark's wife played a vital role, providing emotional support and encouragement. She accompanied him on visits out in public and celebrated his small victories. As Mark faced his triggers, he gained confidence, no longer viewing panic attacks as insurmountable but as manageable episodes that could be navigated with skills and patience.

After several months of therapy, Mark experienced a significant reduction in the frequency and severity of his panic attacks. He reported feeling more willing to engage socially and focus on his work without the constant fear of attack lurking in the background. His story is a testament to the power of persistence, support, and therapeutic intervention.

Notable Individuals with Panic Disorder

Living with panic disorder can feel like navigating a relentless storm—sudden, fierce, and unpredictable. Yet, history shows that even amid profound struggles, resilience and perseverance can lead to extraordinary achievement. Lucille Ball, Stephen King, and Olivia Munn are shining examples that having panic disorder does not have to define one's life or limit their potential.

Lucille Ball: The Queen of Comedy Who Faced Her Fears

Lucille Ball's career remains legendary; her comedic genius brought laughter to millions worldwide. But behind her iconic smile was a woman who battled severe anxiety and panic attacks throughout her career. In her autobiography and interviews, she spoke candidly about her struggle with stage fright and social anxiety, especially during the early days of her career when she was often paralyzed by fear before performances. Her panic episodes made her question whether she could continue in show business, and for years, she tried to hide her fears behind her vibrant persona.

Despite her internal battles, Lucille refused to give up. She sought help in the form of therapy and learned techniques to manage her symptoms—deep breathing, mental grounding, and gradually facing her performance anxieties. Her perseverance paid off;

she persevered through her panic episodes and went on to create one of television's most beloved sitcoms, *I Love Lucy*. Her story teaches us that even the most successful have faced moments of vulnerability and that resilience and seeking support can transform panic into strength.

Stephen King: The Master of Horror Who Confronted His Anxiety

Stephen King, one of the most prolific authors in history, has been candid about his battle with anxiety and panic attacks—especially during times of personal stress and loss. During the height of his career, King experienced debilitating panic episodes that left him feeling helpless and isolated. Despite his success, he often felt overwhelmed by fear, and at times, it affected his productivity and mental health.

King's story is one of persistence. Recognizing his anxiety was a part of him, he sought therapy, developed coping strategies, and used writing as an outlet for his fears and frustrations. He talks openly about the importance of routine, grounding techniques, and seeking help without shame. Today, his books continue to thrill millions, embodying the idea that one can turn personal struggles into powerful expression. Stephen King's journey illustrates that success isn't the absence of anxiety but the courage to face it head-on and keep moving forward.

Olivia Munn: The Actress and Advocate Who Turned Anxiety into Inspiration

Olivia Munn, known for her roles on screen and outspoken advocacy for mental health, openly shares her experience with panic attacks. From a young age, she faced severe social anxiety and panic episodes that made attending social events, auditioning, and even speaking in public daunting tasks. For years, she fought feelings of fear and inadequacy, often feeling isolated by her symptoms.

What makes Olivia's story inspiring is her proactive approach. She sought therapy, learned mindfulness and breathing exercises, and gradually exposed herself to challenging situations. Her determination to not let anxiety define her career and life led her to become an advocate—sharing her journey to normalize mental health struggles and encourage others to seek help. Today, Olivia uses her voice and platform to inspire others facing similar battles, proving that acceptance and resilience can lead to success and fulfillment.

Journaling Prompts

1. Reflect on a recent panic attack: What were the initial symptoms, and what thoughts accompanied them?

2. What specific fears or thoughts often precede a panic episode? How realistic do you think these fears are?

3. Describe how you typically feel after a panic attack passes. What helps you to recover or feel grounded again?

4. How does the fear of having another panic attack influence your daily decisions and activities?

5. Identify a thought pattern related to panic attacks that tends to escalate your anxiety. How might you reframe this thought into something more manageable?

6. Think of a time when you successfully challenged a catastrophic thought. What evidence helped you see a different perspective?

7. How can incorporating positive affirmations before a known trigger help ease anticipatory anxiety?

8. Describe any relaxation techniques or coping strategies you've found helpful in moderating panic symptoms.

9. List the sensations or situations you associate with panic attacks. Which might you confront through exposure therapy?

10. How do you think gradual exposure to feared sensations could help reduce your panic symptoms?

11. Reflect on how structured exposure in a controlled setting—like a therapist's office—can assist in desensitizing panic triggers.

12. Identify any tools or strategies, such as deep breathing or grounding exercises, that help during exposure practices. How do they assist?

13. Consider how your experiences with panic disorder relate to those of the individuals in the case study. What feelings or thoughts does this similarity evoke?

14. How would reducing the frequency and intensity of your panic attacks change your life? What goals or activities could become possible?

15. Who in your life can provide support or encouragement as you work through panic disorder? How might they assist you?

Journaling

Journaling

Chapter Nine

Type 6: Anxious Attachment Style

I HAVE NOTICED IN my own experience that attachment styles have recently become a more popular topic in mainstream society. I see posts and videos about it on social media. People are making books about the topic that are doing well. But it's actually an older subject in the field of psychology. So, what are "attachment styles" anyway? Essentially, the idea is that the way we bond with others is deeply rooted in our early experiences with caregivers. Psychologists John Bowlby and Mary Ainsworth introduced Attachment Theory in the 1960s and 70s, positing that these early bonds form the blueprint for our emotional interactions throughout life. Mary Ainsworth's work further elaborated on the foundation of Attachment Theory through her "Strange Situation" experiments, identifying distinct attachment styles. Understanding these styles provides insight into how individuals connect, love, and sometimes struggle in their adult relationships. Also, please note that I have included a special "cheat sheet" for individuals with anxious attachment at the end of this chapter.

Secure Attachment

Introduction and Development

Secure attachment is considered the ideal style, marking a robust and healthy bond between a child and their caregiver. This attachment develops when caregivers are consistently responsive, nurturing, and attentive to a child's needs. A securely attached child receives comfort when distressed, warmth when nurtured, and validation when exploring their environment.

During a child's early years, secure attachment is fostered through ongoing positive interactions. The caregiver acts as a secure base from which the child can confidently explore the world. When distressed, the child knows they can return to the caregiver for comfort and reassurance. This cycle of trust establishes an internal working model in the child that relationships are dependable and safe.

Manifestation in Adult Relationships

As adults, those with secure attachment typically exhibit confidence in their relationships. They are comfortable with both intimacy and independence, balancing closeness with personal space. Securely attached individuals tend to have fulfilling and stable relationships due to their capacity to trust, communicate effectively, and resolve conflicts amicably. They approach relationships with optimism, seeing them as a source of support and joy rather than vulnerability or fear.

In romantic settings, securely attached adults do not shy away from expressing their needs, desires, or concerns and feel equally equipped to offer support and empathy to their partners. They are likely to choose partners who share similar communication styles and emotional availability, creating a dynamic of mutual respect and shared responsibility.

Emotionally, secure attachment aids individuals in managing stress and anxiety better in relationships. They perceive conflicts as opportunities for growth, rather than seeing them as threats. Thus, the capacity to maintain emotional balance allows securely attached adults to navigate the complexities of relationships with resilience.

When faced with relationship challenges, these individuals are likely to engage in open discussions and seek constructive solutions rather than withdrawing or becoming overly aggressive. This flexibility and emotional awareness foster trust and connectedness, laying the groundwork for successful long-term partnerships.

Avoidant Attachment

Introduction and Development

Avoidant attachment develops when caregivers are emotionally unavailable, physically unavailable, or consistently dismissive of a child's needs. Children who learn that seeking comfort results in rejection, discomfort, or neglect may suppress their emotional needs, turning inward for self-soothing. Through repeated experiences of unresponsive caregiving, a child internalizes the notion that closeness and intimacy result in discomfort or disappointment. This defensive mechanism forms the backdrop for avoidant attachment.

Such children often become self-reliant and detached, a strategy ensuring they are less vulnerable to the caregiver's rejections. They tend to shy away from depending on others, preferring distance and independence over closeness. Over time, this independent façade becomes part of their psychological armor against potential emotional pain.

Manifestation in Adult Relationships

As adults, individuals with avoidant attachment may exhibit a strong desire for independence and self-sufficiency in relationships. Fearing vulnerability, they keep emotional distance even in intimate situations. Avoidantly attached adults often perceive too much intimacy as stifling, leading them to maintain a level of detachment to protect themselves from potential rejection or hurt.

In romantic relationships, this attachment style might manifest as reluctance to express emotions, dismissing the value of close relationships, or avoiding intense commitment. They might struggle to recognize or validate emotional experiences, both in themselves and their partners, appearing emotionally distant or insensitive.

While they may appear confident, avoidantly attached adults often harbor deep-seated insecurities about depending on others. Their self-reliance can be a double-edged sword; it allows for independence but can also isolate them from meaningful connections.

Interventions and Adjustments

If you suspect you have avoidant attachment, you're not alone. As many as 25% of individuals in the general public are estimated to struggle with the symptoms of avoidant attachment: balancing independence and intimacy, often feeling discomfort when relationships become too close. Fortunately, there are practical techniques to help foster healthier relationship dynamics.

First, practice self-awareness through journaling. Reflect on moments when you withdrew or felt uncomfortable, helping you recognize patterns and underlying fears about dependence or vulnerability. Pair this with mindfulness exercises—such as focused breathing or body scans—that cultivate a calm, present awareness of emotions. This helps reduce the impulse to shut down when intimacy feels overwhelming.

Gradual exposure is key. Start by sharing small personal details or expressing needs with trusted friends or partners. Over time, increase emotional sharing at your own pace, reinforcing that closeness doesn't threaten your independence. Complement this with positive self-talk and challenging beliefs like "Trusting others will make me lose myself." Instead, try affirmations like "I can be close while maintaining my independence."

Developing communication skills—asserting needs clearly and listening actively—can deepen bonds without triggering fears. Building relationships with supportive, patient individuals provides safety for gradually softening your guarded stance. Remember, setting healthy boundaries and prioritizing self-care reinforce your autonomy while still engaging meaningfully with others.

Finally, working with a therapist trained in attachment-based approaches can help you explore fears, process past experiences, and develop long-term patterns of secure relating. Change takes time, so celebrate small steps and stay patient with yourself.

Anxious Attachment

Introduction and Development

Anxious attachment develops when caregiving is inconsistent, unpredictable, or overly intrusive. Children with this attachment style might experience caregivers who alternate between responsive and neglectful behaviors, leaving the child uncertain about how their needs will be met. This inconsistency creates anxiety, as the child fails to develop a reliable model for how relationships function.

As children, those with anxious attachment find themselves in a cycle of seeking closeness, feeling insecure when unattainable, and thus clinging to their caregiver to gain reassurance. The child learns to become hyper-vigilant to any signs of threat or withdrawal, craving continual validation to affirm their worth and relational security.

Manifestation in Adult Relationships

In adulthood, anxious attachment often presents as a strong need for closeness and reassurance, coupled with heightened sensitivity to perceived threats to the relationship. Adults with anxious attachment may feel a pervasive uncertainty about their partner's feelings, leading to fears of abandonment and rejection. This can result in behaviors such as clinging, dependency, or frequent demands for assurance from their partners.

Anxiously attached individuals often read too deeply into their partner's actions, interpreting neutral or ambiguous behavior as signs of disinterest or unfaithfulness. This hypersensitivity can lead to conflict, as they may express their fears in ways that appear controlling or overly demanding, seeking constant validation to soothe their insecurities.

In romantic relationships, these individuals might find themselves in a cycle of seeking closeness, feeling momentarily reassured, then experiencing a return of insecurity and doubt. Their fear of losing the relationship may drive them to over-analyze or catastrophize situations, which can be taxing both for themselves and their partners.

Interventions and Adjustments

If you recognize traits of anxious attachment—such as fearing rejection, needing constant reassurance, or feeling insecure in relationships—you may belong to the estimated 20% of the population that has developed this attachment style. These feelings often stem from early experiences where caregivers were inconsistent, unavailable, or overbearing, creating a deep-seated fear of abandonment.

The good news is that anxious attachment is reversible with intentional effort. The following is a short guide for helping individuals to overcome their anxious attachment style:

Self-awareness is the foundation of change. Journaling can help individuals identify triggers and recognize patterns of anxious thought. For instance, note moments when you felt particularly anxious or needed reassurance, probing the emotions underlying these feelings. Recognizing cyclic self-talk like "I'm not good enough" or "They will leave me" enables the breaking down of anxiety-inducing thoughts.

Enhancing self-esteem involves recognizing personal worth and developing a positive self-image independent of relationship status. Setting and achieving small, personal goals unrelated to the relationship—for example, pursuing a hobby or developing a new skill—can boost confidence. Acknowledging personal accomplishments, no matter how minor, fosters a sense of individual identity separate from attachment needs.

Cognitive Behavioral Therapy (CBT) is particularly effective in modifying negative thought patterns. Techniques include challenging irrational beliefs, such as "If they don't text me back, they don't care." Cognitive restructuring involves weighing evidence for and against such beliefs and developing alternative, more balanced views like "They may be busy, have their phone turned off, or something else. It's not automatically a sign of abandonment." The focus is on reframing interpretations of partners' behaviors to reduce dependency on validation.

Developing mindfulness skills helps combat impulsive reactions to anxious thoughts. Practices such as mindful breathing or meditation increase awareness of the present moment, reducing the tendency to catastrophize future events. This can be practiced by setting aside time each day for meditation, focusing on the breath, and observing thoughts without judgment. Over time, this builds resilience against emotional storms and refines emotional regulation skills.

Learning to communicate needs assertively and positively is crucial. Anxiously attached individuals might avoid expressing needs for fear of burdensomeness. Role-play scenarios that involve seeking clarity or reassurance without becoming confrontational. Establish clear, mutual communication with partners about boundaries and individual needs. Agree on signals or words to use if someone feels overwhelmed, ensuring both partners can express comfort and security within the relationship.

Fostering secure attachment involves the ability to be vulnerable. Discuss fears openly with trustworthy partners, finding common ground for understanding each other's perspectives. Empathy and active listening are powerful, allowing both partners to feel heard and validated without perpetuating a cycle of reassurance-seeking. Encourage partner participation in relationship building, including completing shared tasks or creating common goals.

Working with a therapist familiar with attachment styles can provide deeper insight. Therapies like Emotionally Focused Therapy (EFT) or Attachment-Based Therapy focus on transforming attachment patterns and developing healthier relational dynamics. Therapists help individuals recognize core issues driving anxiety and develop adaptive coping mechanisms in safe, nurturing environments.

Transitioning from anxious to secure attachment entails consistent, incremental practice. Reinforce security by recalling positive moments in the relationship when anxiety subsides and connection feels genuine. Building secure patterns encompasses tasks like integrating self-soothing rituals—taking a warm bath, journaling accolades—into daily routines, shifting focus to self-reliant, positive practices.

Disorganized Attachment

Introduction and Development

Disorganized attachment often emerges from a childhood environment marked by chaos, abuse, or unresolved trauma. Caregivers in these settings might display frightening or unpredictable behavior, making it difficult for the child to develop a coherent strategy for receiving comfort or protection. This confusion leads to a lack of consistent coping mechanisms and attachment strategies.

Children with disorganized attachment find themselves caught between seeking security and fearing their caregiver's presence. This leads to disorientation and uncertainty about relationships, as their source of comfort simultaneously becomes a source of fear. They might exhibit behaviors that seem erratic or contradictory, such as approaching a caregiver only to retreat in fear.

Over time, this attachment style results in difficulty forming a stable sense of self or understanding where to find safety, leaving lasting impacts on their relational and emotional development.

Manifestation in Adult Relationships

In adult relationships, disorganized attachment can lead to a complex mix of fear and desire for closeness. Adults with this style might oscillate between seeking intimacy and engaging in behaviors that sabotage closeness, often without understanding their motivations. They may genuinely desire closeness yet feel overwhelmed by the fear or confusion it brings.

This attachment style often results in tumultuous relationships, marked by instability and an underlying sense of chaos. Individuals might struggle with trust and exhibit both clingy and distancing behaviors, complicating their ability to sustain healthy, secure bonds. Emotional regulation can be a challenge, leading to intense emotions and reactions that may seem bewildering to both the individual and their partners.

Interventions and Adjustments

If you relate to disorganized attachment, you're likely caught in a confusing inner struggle—pulling toward closeness but also pulling away out of fear or mistrust. This attachment style often develops from childhood experiences marked by trauma, neglect, or inconsistent caregiving, leaving a tangled web of conflicting feelings about trust and safety. The good news is that, with gentle effort and practical strategies, you can begin to untangle those knots and foster healthier, more secure connections.

One powerful starting point is cultivating greater self-awareness. Regularly reflecting on your feelings during moments of intimacy or conflict can help you recognize patterns—perhaps noticing moments when you push away because of fear, or when you seek reassurance but then doubt your partner's intentions. Journaling these experiences can clarify your internal landscape and make it easier to identify triggers.

When feelings of anxiety or disorientation start to surge, grounding techniques such as deep breathing or focusing on your senses can calm the flood and give you room to choose a deliberate response rather than reacting impulsively. These tools help create a sense of internal safety, which is essential for building trust over time.

Learning to identify and label your emotions—whether fear, shame, or confusion—further reduces their power. This process allows you to speak more honestly about your needs and fears in your relationship, gradually building open communication. Sharing your feelings with your partner in small, manageable steps can help you develop trust and comfort in vulnerability.

Establishing clear boundaries and respecting your limits is equally important. Think about what safe space feels like for you and communicate that to your partner. Consistency and predictability in setting and maintaining boundaries foster a sense of safety that encourages trust to grow.

Working with a therapist trained in attachment-focused or trauma-informed approaches can further facilitate healing. Techniques like internal parts work or trauma processing help integrate conflicting feelings, strengthening your sense of internal safety and stability. Ultimately, practicing kindness and self-compassion along the way—reminding yourself that healing takes time—is key. Over time, these intentional efforts can help you build the secure, loving relationships you deserve.

Separation Anxiety Disorder

In the section of the DSM-5 dedicated to anxiety disorders, there is a disorder that is called "Separation Anxiety Disorder," which addresses children who fail to securely attach to their caregivers. I should point out that not all children who fail to securely attach to caregivers have this disorder. Despite what you might assume, this is not a disorder that children primarily deal with. For many individuals, the age of onset begins in late adolescence or even in their 20s.

Separation Anxiety Disorder (SAD) is a complex condition that, while often associated with children, can affect individuals across the lifespan. It represents a deep-rooted fear of being separated from significant attachment figures, leading to distress that is disproportionate to the situation. Understanding the nuances of this disorder can shed light on its impact and offer pathways to effective management.

DSM-5 Symptoms of Separation Anxiety Disorder

According to the Diagnostic and Statistical Manual of Mental Disorders, Fifth Edition (DSM-5), Separation Anxiety Disorder is marked by excessive fear or anxiety concerning separation from home or attachment figures **(criteria A)**. This anxiety is characterized by several key points:

1. **Recurrent Excessive Distress:** Individuals experience significant distress when

anticipating or being away from home or major attachment figures. This often manifests as panic attacks or extreme reactions in the face of actual or anticipated separation.

2. **Persistent and Excessive Worry About Losing Major Attachment Figures:** The anxiety often includes fears of losing these figures to illness, disaster, or tragedy, resulting in intrusive thoughts and compulsive behaviors aimed at preventing separation.

3. **Persistent and Excessive Worry About Experiencing an Untoward Event that Causes Separation from a Major Attachment Figure:** This includes fears of getting lost, being kidnapped, having an accident, or becoming ill. It can also manifest as intrusive thoughts and compulsive behaviors.

4. **Reluctance or Refusal to Go Out:** This includes hesitation to leave home for school, work, or other activities due to fear of separation, which can interfere with social, academic, or occupational functioning.

5. **Persistent and Excessive Fear of or Reluctance About Being Alone or Without Major Attachment Figures at Home or in Other Settings:** These fears can lead to avoidance behaviors (resisting going to school or work), physical symptoms (headaches and nausea), nightmares, difficulty sleeping, and impairment in daily functioning.

6. **Persistent Reluctance or Refusal to Sleep Away From Home or to Go to Sleep Without Being Near a Major Attachment Figure:** Some of these manifestations include refusing to go to sleep unless a parent is present, repeatedly waking up during the night and seeking out the parent, or even refusing to sleep in their own bed.

7. **Repeated Nightmares Involving the Theme of Separation:** This manifestation is rather common, with the content often revolving around themes of separation, loss, or harm coming to the attachment figure.

8. **Repeated Complaints of Physical Symptoms When Separation From**

Major Attachment Figures Occurs or is Anticipated: Symptoms include headaches, stomachaches, nausea, and vomiting.

To meet the diagnostic criteria, these symptoms must last at least four weeks in children or six months in adults **(criteria B)** and cause significant distress or impair functioning **(criteria C)**. Also, the disturbance must not be better explained by another mental disorder **(criteria D)**.

Prevalence and Demographics

Separation Anxiety Disorder affects about 4-5% of children, making it one of the most common anxiety disorders in this demographic. Interestingly, it's not exclusive to childhood; approximately 1-2% of adults also experience this disorder. While many children with separation anxiety grow out of it, some symptoms can carry into adulthood, manifesting in difficulties coping with separations at work or in personal relationships.

The disorder does not affect all demographics equally. It is slightly more common in females than males in both childhood and adulthood. Cultural factors can influence its expression; for instance, in societies where familial interdependence is emphasized, the disorder may manifest differently.

Development of Separation Anxiety Disorder

Separation Anxiety Disorder often develops in early childhood, typically between the ages of 3 and 14, aligning with developmental stages when children begin attending school. This period is crucial for establishing independence from caregivers, and separation anxiety is considered part of normal development until it becomes excessive or persists beyond age-appropriate levels.

The disorder can be triggered or exacerbated by stressful life events such as parental divorce, moving to a new place, starting at a new school, or the loss of a loved one. In response to these changes, children—and sometimes adults—can experience heightened attachment behaviors as strategies to maintain security and minimize perceived threats.

The development of the disorder is also influenced by genetic and environmental factors. A family history of anxiety disorders, particularly in first-degree relatives, can increase susceptibility. Additionally, parenting styles play a substantial role; overprotective or anxious parenting can inadvertently reinforce a child's anxiety by limiting their exposure to independent experiences, preventing the formation of coping mechanisms necessary for confident separation.

Contributing Factors

Several factors can intensify separation anxiety symptoms, turning manageable apprehensions into significant disturbances.

Inconsistent Parenting: Swinging between permissive and authoritative styles may confuse children, fostering insecurity about when and where they feel safe, further entrenching avoidance behaviors.

Traumatic Experiences: Situations involving abrupt or traumatic separations—such as accidents, sudden relocations, or family emergencies—can intensify separation anxiety, making restoration of stability more difficult.

Environmental Stressors: Significant changes, such as a pandemic or economic downturn, that reshape daily routines can heighten anxiety levels. These stressors place additional burdens on individuals who already fear separation, especially when they complicate access to support networks.

Co-existing Mental Health Conditions: Depressive disorders or other anxiety disorders often coexist with separation anxiety, amplifying its symptoms and complicating treatment outcomes.

School and Social Dynamics: Bullying, academic pressures, or social exclusion can worsen anxiety, particularly in children, leading them to cling to known comforts (such as family) and resist stepping into potentially hostile or demanding environments.

Addressing separation anxiety disorder involves understanding its roots and recognizing the factors that intensify it. Effective treatment can alleviate symptoms and foster resilience through a combination of Cognitive Behavioral Therapy (CBT), Exposure Therapy, and, when necessary, pharmaceutical intervention. Here, we explore tailored techniques and strategies that can empower individuals to conquer their anxiety.

Cognitive Behavioral Therapy (CBT)

CBT offers a toolkit for individuals with separation anxiety, transforming thought patterns and behaviors that exacerbate fear. One practical technique within CBT is cognitive restructuring, which involves helping individuals identify and alter distorted beliefs about separation. For instance, if a child fears something catastrophic will happen when they're away from their parents, the therapist guides them to challenge these beliefs, focusing on evidence of past successful separations without adverse outcomes. This cognitive shift alleviates anxiety by reinforcing the safety of the situation.

In addition, CBT often incorporates teaching coping skills such as problem-solving and self-soothing. A child or adult with separation anxiety may benefit from learning specific techniques to calm themselves, such as breathing exercises or visualization methods. Guided imagery allows them to picture themselves in a safe space, away from home, effectively reducing panic symptoms manifested by distant travel or solo activities.

Role-playing exercises are another CBT strategy that empowers individuals to practice separation in a controlled, supportive environment. For instance, a child might practice saying goodbye at the door with a therapist acting as a parent, rehearsing positive parting routines to reframe goodbyes as a normal, reassuring ritual rather than a stress-inducing experience.

Exposure Therapy

Exposure therapy targets the behavioral aspects of separation anxiety by gradually reducing avoidance behavior through controlled exposure to separation scenarios. A hierarchal approach is commonly used, starting with minor separations and progressing to longer ones. For example, a child might first practice staying in a different room from their parent for short periods and gradually build to spending time at a friend's house alone.

Systematic desensitization is a key exposure strategy, where therapists pair exposure exercises with relaxation techniques. If an adult struggles with anxiety about leaving a loved one at home, exposure exercises might involve taking short trips alone while using relaxation techniques learned in therapy to soothe any rising panic.

Virtual reality environments are increasingly utilized within exposure therapy to simulate separation scenarios. This technology can offer adults struggling to leave a spouse or children a way to experience separation in a highly controlled, customizable setup, allowing them to practice coping mechanisms before facing situations in real life.

Pharmaceutical Options

Pharmaceutical intervention, while not always necessary, can complement therapy for individuals with severe separation anxiety, providing relief from acute symptoms and allowing therapy to take hold more effectively. Selective Serotonin Reuptake Inhibitors (SSRIs), such as fluoxetine (Prozac) or sertraline (Zoloft), are commonly prescribed. They can help stabilize mood and reduce anxiety by increasing serotonin levels, leading to decreased distress about separation scenarios.

For short-term relief, particularly during periods of heightened anxiety, short-acting benzodiazepines may be used with caution. However, their long-term use is typically avoided to prevent dependency. Careful medical oversight ensures that medication is appropriately integrated into a broader treatment plan.

The Path Forward

Effective treatment of Separation Anxiety Disorder involves more than symptom management. Effective helpers seek to empower individuals to develop skills and resilience, providing them with tools to handle separation with confidence.

By balancing CBT and Exposure Therapy with strategic medication use when necessary, individuals learn to trust in their capacity to handle independence, transforming separation from a source of distress into an aspect of personal growth. Encouraging supportive environments—where open communication, patience, and empathy are prioritized—facilitates progress, ensuring that those affected by separation anxiety can realize their potential and navigate their world with peace and confidence.

For caregivers and individuals alike, consistent practice, reinforcement of skills, and gentle encouragement are vital. Over time, with the right strategies and support, separation anxiety can become manageable, allowing individuals to embrace independence and the growth it offers, ultimately fostering a life rich with connection and fulfillment.

Separation Anxiety Disorder in Culture

Separation Anxiety Disorder (SAD) in its clinical sense hasn't often been explicitly documented in historical figures, largely because the formal diagnosis is relatively modern. However, historical accounts and biographical analyses sometimes suggest behaviors consistent with separation anxiety, though they are primarily speculative.

In terms of contemporary public figures, specific instances of Separation Anxiety Disorder haven't been prominently disclosed, perhaps due to the personal nature of the condition and the general stigma historically associated with mental health issues. However, public awareness and acceptance have increased, leading more individuals to talk openly about various mental health challenges.

It's important to recognize that public disclosure about specific mental health diagnoses, particularly one such as Separation Anxiety Disorder, which might still carry certain societal misunderstandings, is limited. Instead, many individuals, including public figures, choose to speak about anxiety more generally, often encompassing a range of experiences and symptoms without specifying a distinct subtype like SAD.

For those interested in exploring narratives of separation anxiety, literature, and biographical accounts provide nuanced examples of prominent figures experiencing anxiety in various forms, though the link to SAD might not be directly addressed.

Case Study: Little Lily — Navigating the Fear of Leaving Home

Lily is a 9-year-old girl living in a suburban neighborhood with her parents and her younger brother. From the outside, Lily appears cheerful and bright, excelling in school and engaging readily with her friends. However, her parents have become increasingly concerned about her intense fear of separation from them, which has grown over the past six months.

Lily's father recalls that, initially, her fears manifested as reluctance to go to school. She would cling tightly to him at drop-off, crying and begging to stay home. But her separation anxiety soon extended beyond school drop-offs to everyday activities. She refused to stay over at friends' houses, stating fears that something bad might happen if she's away from her parents. Even in her own home, she experiences panic when her parents leave her sight, often requesting that they stay in the same room with her or sit nearby.

Lily describes her distress in vivid terms. She reports feeling "scared that something will happen to Mom or Dad—like they'll get hurt or never come back." Her worries intensify at bedtime; she insists that her parents stay until she falls asleep and frequently wakes crying during the night, fearing she might be alone or that her parents might leave her in the night. She often experiences physical symptoms—stomachaches, headaches, and difficulty breathing—especially when she anticipates separation.

Her parents express frustration—they want her to participate in social activities and develop independence, yet her fears keep her tied to their side. They notice that Lily is increasingly withdrawn from school events and extracurricular activities, fearing that any outing might lead to separation anxiety episodes or disaster. They have taken her to pediatricians and psychologists to rule out medical issues, and while medical causes have been eliminated, Lily's fears continue.

During the initial assessment, Lily's psychologist, Dr. Lin, noted that her symptoms persisted for over four months and caused significant impairment in her daily functioning—limiting social interactions, school attendance, and family routines. She frequently expressed intolerance for being separated, and her worries included fears about losing her parents, being abandoned, or experiencing harm when apart.

Based on her history and symptoms, Dr. Lin diagnosed Lily with Separation Anxiety Disorder, as outlined in the DSM-5. The diagnosis fit, with Lily's excessive fears of separation, persistent worry, physical symptoms, and avoidance behavior having lasted longer than four weeks and causing marked distress.

The treatment plan centered around gentle, child-appropriate cognitive-behavioral strategies combined with family support. Dr. Lin explained that her goal was to help Lily gradually build confidence in her ability to manage separation, without overwhelming her. Therapy sessions involved teaching Lily relaxation methods—deep breathing and grounding exercises—to manage her physical symptoms. The therapist also worked with Lily to identify and challenge her catastrophic thoughts, such as "If I'm away from Mom and Dad, something really bad will happen."

A key component was exposure work. Initially, Lily practiced brief separations within the safety of her home—such as her parents leaving her with a trusted caregiver for five minutes while she played. These exercises were followed by praise and reassurance, emphasizing that she was safe and that her feelings of fear, though real, were manageable. Over time, these separations extended to trips to her grandparents' house, short walks around the block, and eventually a weekend stay at her cousin's house, always supported by her parents and her therapist.

In addition, her parents learned ways to support her without reinforcing her fears—such as praising her efforts for facing separations, maintaining clear and consistent routines, and providing reassurance that her feelings are valid but manageable. They worked on not overly reassuring her or dismissing her fears, instead validating her emotions and encouraging independence at a comfortable pace.

Over the course of several months, Lily's anxiety reduced significantly. She reported feeling more confident about being away from her parents for short periods and started participating in school activities and playdates again. Her stomachaches and crying episodes decreased, and she was able to fall asleep with less staged reassurance. Her parents felt relieved, and Lily was proud of herself for confronting her fears gradually.

Anxious Attachment Cheat Sheet
Daily Practices to Alleviate Attachment Anxiety

1. *Exercise:* get outside and get some fresh air and sunshine. Go for a walk or a jog. Extra points if you get into the gym and do some resistance training.

2. *Mindful Breathing:* also known to some as the practice of "meditation." Put on some relaxing music. Clear your mind. Observe your thoughts non-judgmentally for 5 minutes.

3. *Gratitude Journaling:* write down three things you are grateful for each day to shift focus from perceived threats to positivity.

4. *Positive Self-Affirmations:* reflect on how you are becoming the person you want to become a little more every day. Think about the things you like the most about yourself. How many can you list?

When Disaster Strikes: Something Has Triggered Your Attachment Anxiety... Now What?

1. *Remember Your CBT Training:* are you catastrophizing? Are you engaging in mind reading? What about future predicting? All of the above? Remember that we are all individuals, and just because someone in the past left you or mistreated you doesn't mean that everyone will.

2. *Have You Exercised Today:* one of the things that can really take the edge off of your anxious energy is to go move around a lot. You will probably feel at least some sense of release.

3. *Try Box Breathing:* remember the technique from chapter 2 about box breathing? Now is a good time to put it to the test. Give your brain and your body a few minutes to come back to baseline.

4. *Remember That Your Basic Self-Worth Is Not At Stake:* no one is perfect and no one should expect you to be. No one can remove your inherent worth by leaving you.

Journaling Prompts

1. When you think about separation or being apart from loved ones, what specific fears or thoughts come up?

2. Do you experience physical symptoms—like stomach aches, headaches, or racing heart—when you think about being separated? How intense are these sensations?

3. How often do you avoid situations that require being away from important attachment figures? What patterns do you notice?

4. How does your fear of separation affect your daily routines, work, or social interactions?

5. Do you tend to seek closeness and reassurance excessively, or do you prefer to keep emotional distance? How does this affect your relationships?

6. When you feel upset or anxious, do you tend to ask for reassurance or try to handle it alone? What does that say about your attachment style?

7. Think of a time when you felt safe or secure in a relationship. What behaviors or feelings contributed to that sense of safety?

8. When conflicts or disagreements occur in your relationships, do you withdraw or become clingy? How do you think this pattern developed?

9. What coping strategies have you tried when feeling anxious about separation? Which ones have helped, and which ones haven't?

10. How might relaxation techniques like deep breathing, grounding, or visualization help you manage separation anxiety?

11. What small steps could you take to gradually increase your independence while still feeling supported?

12. How can you practice validating your feelings without letting anxiety control your actions?

13. Do you see similarities between your experiences and the person in the case study? What feelings or thoughts does this evoke?

14. What lessons can you learn from the case study about overcoming fears and building trust?

15. How might you respond differently in situations where you feel overwhelmed by separation or loss?

Journaling

Journaling

Chapter Ten

Type 7: Existential Anxiety

Congratulations on making it to chapter ten! We are drawing near to the end now, and this chapter marks a definite shift in content. The next few chapters are moving away from DSM-5 anxiety disorders, shifting to miscellaneous topics that are important for understanding anxiety and how we deal with it effectively. This chapter's focus will be Existential Anxiety and how it often manifests itself in our lives. I have chosen to use the concept of "midlife crisis" as a kind of metaphor or template for an "existential crisis," since the midlife crisis metaphor is well represented in modern culture.

I want to start off this chapter by introducing you, briefly, to some of the great contributors to the field of existential philosophy and psychology. I will warn you that if you explore some of the works of these philosophers by reading their original texts, you may find them to be a bit dry. In all honesty, I have never experienced more moments of "what did I just read?" while exploring this topic than just about any other subject I have read in my life. Frankly, some of the concepts in existentialism can seem pedantic, pretentious, or downright confusing. Yet, for all the negatives, this branch of philosophy has some of the most rich insights about life as a human that you will find in any area of literature. So, let's start with a brief overview of some of the great contributors to existentialist thought.

Exploring Existentialism: Major Contributors to the Philosophy

Existentialism is a powerful philosophical movement that focuses on individual freedom, choice, and the quest for meaning in life. It emerged during the nineteenth and twentieth centuries, reminding us that our lives are shaped by the choices we make and the authenticity with which we live. Here are some of the major contributors to this field.

Søren Kierkegaard: The Father of Existentialism

Søren Kierkegaard, a Danish philosopher, is often called the "father of existentialism." He emphasized the idea that life is a series of personal choices, and our true essence isn't given to us but is something we create through those choices. Kierkegaard introduced the notion of the "leap of faith," emphasizing that when rationality can't explain everything, faith prevails. He encouraged individuals to embrace their unique existence and personal beliefs rather than conforming to societal norms.

Friedrich Nietzsche: Questioning Morality

Friedrich Nietzsche, a German philosopher, challenged traditional ideas of morality and religion. He famously declared that "God is dead," suggesting that societal progress had diminished the role of religious beliefs. Nietzsche introduced the concept of the Übermensch, or "Overman," urging us to transcend conventional values and create our own meaning and morals. His philosophy challenges us to embrace individuality, creativity, and personal growth, rather than passively accepting inherited beliefs.

Jean-Paul Sartre: Freedom and Responsibility

Jean-Paul Sartre, a French philosopher, gave us the idea that "existence precedes essence," which means that a person exists first, and only through their actions and choices does that person define their own nature or "essence." Sartre believed that true freedom comes with the weight of responsibility, as every decision shapes our character and world. He famously said, "We are condemned to be free," highlighting the sometimes daunting yet liberating nature of making choices that define our lives.

Viktor Frankl: Finding Meaning

Viktor Frankl, an Austrian neurologist and psychiatrist, survived the horror of Nazi concentration camps and profoundly impacted existential thought, particularly through his psychological approach known as *logotherapy*. Frankl emphasized the "will to meaning," the belief that our primary drive in life is not pleasure or power, but finding a meaningful purpose. Through his experiences, he concluded that even in the harshest circumstances, we can find meaning in suffering and that personal responsibility empowers us to create our own life's purpose.

Albert Camus: Embracing the Absurd

Albert Camus, a French-Algerian philosopher, focused on the conflict between our desire for meaning and the indifferent universe—a concept he called "the absurd." In his essay *The Myth of Sisyphus*, Camus illustrated this by depicting the Greek myth of Sisyphus, a man condemned to eternally roll a boulder uphill, only for it to roll back down. Camus argued that, despite life's absurdity, we should embrace it, find joy in defiance, and "revolt" against meaninglessness.

Martin Heidegger: Being and Time

Martin Heidegger, a German philosopher, introduced the concept of "Being-in-the-world" as a way to explore how humans exist authentically. His work focused on examining the nature of being and time from a personal perspective. Heidegger proposed that individuals often live inauthentically, influenced by societal pressures rather than their true selves. He urged awareness of our finite lives to prompt genuine existence and self-discovery.

Each of these thinkers offers unique insights into the nature of existence, challenging us to reflect on our beliefs, confront our mortality, and consider the essence of what it means to live genuinely. While their ideas may stem from heavier philosophical thought, at their core, they urge us to embrace freedom, define our life's purpose, and live authentically.

The Heart of Existentialism: Exploring Its Main Themes

Existentialism is a philosophical movement that challenges us to think deeply about what it means to live a genuine life. It emphasizes personal responsibility, freedom, and the search for meaning in a world that often feels unpredictable or indifferent. While the ideas can seem heavy, they offer valuable insights into how we can find purpose and authenticity amid life's uncertainties. Let's explore some of the core themes that run through existentialist thought.

Freedom and Responsibility

At the core of existentialism is the idea that humans are free. We are not born with a fixed purpose or destiny handed to us; instead, we have the power—and the burden—to shape our own lives. Every choice we make defines who we are. But with this freedom comes responsibility: we are accountable for our decisions and their consequences. This can be both empowering and daunting.

For example, imagine standing at a crossroads—one path leads to a career you love, while the other might offer more money but less fulfillment. Choice seems simple, but existentialists remind us that we carry the weight for what follows. We cannot blame society, circumstances, or genetics entirely; ultimately, we decide what kind of person we want to be. This realization encourages authenticity—living according to our true values—despite social pressures to conform.

The Absurd and Meaning

One of the most profound themes in existentialism is the "absurd" — the idea that humans constantly search for meaning in life, but the universe offers no inherent answer. It's as if you're trying to read a book that has no ending; your desire for purpose clashes with a universe that appears silent or indifferent. This confrontation with life's absurdity can produce feelings of despair, but philosophers like Albert Camus suggest it's also an opportunity.

Camus argues that, instead of despairing, we should accept life's absurd nature and live passionately anyway. Like Sisyphus, condemned to push a boulder uphill for eternity, we can find joy in rebellion, in creating our own meaning despite life's apparent lack of it. This act of defiance—of choosing to live fully in the face of absurdity—is a key way to find authentic purpose.

Authenticity and Inauthenticity

Existentialism stresses the importance of authenticity—living in a way that is true to oneself—rather than conforming to societal expectations or adopting a false identity. When people act out of fear of judgment or follow prescribed roles without introspection, they live in "bad faith," a term coined by Jean-Paul Sartre.

For instance, a person working a job they dislike just to meet societal standards is living inauthentically. An authentic life involves embracing personal choices, acknowledging fears, and acting in alignment with one's deepest values. Though challenging, authenticity grants a profound sense of freedom and integrity.

Isolation and Alienation

A recurring theme is human loneliness—even when we are surrounded by others. Individual existence can feel isolating because each person experiences life from their own subjective perspective. This alienation becomes pronounced when people suppress their true feelings or hide behind masks to please others.

Existentialists urge us to confront this loneliness and accept our mortality—recognizing that life is fleeting. Doing so can deepen our appreciation for authentic relationships and lead us to live more fully, knowing that each moment is precious and limited.

Death and the Search for Meaning

Finally, death is an unavoidable part of life that confronts us with our mortality. Many existentialists believe that awareness of death should inspire us to live authentically. Facing mortality forces us to ask: What truly matters? What legacy do I want to leave?

What Is Existential Anxiety?

Many people experience a strange, sometimes uncomfortable feeling when they think about the big questions of life: "What is my purpose?" "What happens after we die?" or "Why am I here?" These thoughts can trigger feelings of worry, fear, or even helplessness. This kind of deep, reflective nervousness is often called *existential anxiety*, and it is something that most psychologists and therapists say is a normal part of being human.

Unlike everyday fears—like being afraid of heights, spiders, or failing a test—existential anxiety is rooted in the way we think about life itself. It's about our understanding that life is uncertain, that we will one day grow old and die, and that life doesn't always come with clear, easy answers. It's a natural response to recognizing that, at some point, everyone faces the big questions we can't fully solve or control.

Why Do People Feel This Way?

When we fully realize our mortality—that we are finite and that death is inevitable—it can make us feel small or vulnerable. However, rather than scare us, it should remind us that life is precious and limited. Sometimes, this awareness pushes us to think about what really matters: our relationships, our passions, and how we want to spend our days. For many, this realization is motivating. It encourages us to live authentically, pursue meaningful work, and cherish our loved ones.

However, for others, pondering these questions without understanding or support can lead to anxiety. The feelings may become overwhelming, and some people might get stuck in worries about whether their lives are meaningful enough or whether they're afraid of dying alone or unloved. When these fears become intense and persistent, they can interfere with daily life, leading to feelings of despair or depression.

Psychologists call this "existential anxiety" because it's tied to our awareness of life's biggest mysteries. It's not a disorder in itself but a normal human emotion that can become problematic if it leads to feelings of hopelessness or excessive fear. However, even these emotions can serve a purpose, if they motivate us to change our lives in some kind of transformative way that brings us satisfaction from resolving our existential crisis.

How Is It Different from Other Types of Anxiety?

Most everyday worries are about specific things—failing a test, missing a meeting, or falling ill. But existential anxiety is about broad, fundamental concerns about life itself. It's not about one specific fear; rather, it's about questioning whether life has meaning, dread related to mortality, or fears about the unknown.

For example, imagine feeling uneasy when you realize life is fleeting and that someday, you will die. That feeling—sometimes called "death anxiety"—is a common part of existential anxiety. Many people find this awareness unsettling because it challenges their need for certainty and control over their life.

But existential anxiety isn't necessarily negative. It can be a catalyst for personal growth if we learn to face these fears thoughtfully. When we accept the uncertainties of life—acknowledging that nobody has all the answers—we often find more peace and a deeper appreciation for the present moment.

Is It Normal to Feel Like This?

Absolutely. The philosopher and psychologist Viktor Frankl, who survived the Holocaust, believed that grappling with life's ultimate questions is part of being human. Many mental health experts say that some degree of existential anxiety is universal, especially when we face difficult life transitions, loss, or big decisions. It's a sign that you're engaging deeply with your life and its meaning.

The key is not to eliminate these feelings but to understand and accept them. Rather than run from the questions, you can view them as an invitation to discover what truly matters to you and to live authentically.

When Does It Become a Problem?

While some existential anxiety leads to growth, it can become harmful when it causes overwhelming fear, paralysis, or despair. If thoughts about death, meaning, or the future prevent you from functioning—making everyday activities difficult, leading to avoidance, or fostering hopelessness—then it's helpful to seek support.

People may experience this in different ways. Some might obsessively worry about death, others might feel a sense of emptiness or meaninglessness, and some may develop anxiety about future uncertainties, such as economic stability or health concerns.

Case Study: David's Crossroads — Navigating the Midlife Crisis

David had always considered himself an average man. As a middle-aged marketing executive, he'd built a comfortable life—steady job, a suburban home, and a loving family.

Yet, somewhere in the last few years, a restless unease began to gnaw at him. It wasn't simply the fatigue of routines or the pressures of work; it was a deeper, more unsettling feeling—an unease that he couldn't quite shake.

David's mornings now felt heavier. Even when he awoke in his warm bed beside his wife, a sense of emptiness persisted. His job no longer brought him joy, and increasingly, he found himself questioning the purpose of his work and life. "Is this really all there is?" he would wonder silently, staring at the ceiling after tossing and turning all night. The vibrant dreams of his youth, filled with ambitions and passions, seemed distant now, replaced by a fog of stagnation.

Outside, the world appeared to be rushing forward—new technologies, changing social norms, and an endless stream of headlines that screamed about climate change, political upheaval, and societal chaos. David felt like he was caught between a desire to engage and a deep fear of facing the reality that all these external changes signified a deeper, personal crisis: what is the purpose of it all?

He began to notice that friends and colleagues seemed to be caught in the same web—some were chasing material success, others were retreating into hobbies or into silence, trying to avoid the gnawing questions about meaning and mortality. David, however, felt trapped. His business accomplishments seemed hollow, his relationships with his wife and children sometimes strained by his unspoken grumblings and episodes of despair.

One weekend, while sitting alone in his study, surrounded by work notebooks, family photos, and books he no longer felt excited about, David finally allowed himself to fully confront what he'd been avoiding. The feeling was like a shadow stretching over him—an acknowledgement that perhaps, deep down, he was facing a crisis of existence. Was this all life was meant to be? Had he simply coasted through years, avoiding the uncomfortable truths?

Over the next few months, David began to seek help. He found a counselor who gently guided him through his feelings of emptiness and doubt. They discussed what many philosophers and psychologists describe as an "existential crisis"—a period when fundamental questions about life's meaning and death surface, often triggered by life transitions that can happen in midlife.

In his therapy, David learned that his feelings were rooted in what existentialists and psychologists call *existential anxiety*—the deep-seated awareness of mortality, freedom, and the fleeting nature of life. He was confronting the fact that his time was limited, and the question emerged—what is the true purpose of his life? His fear of insignificance and the realization that he was living on autopilot created a whirlwind of emotional turmoil.

He was encouraged to explore his core values—what truly mattered to him beyond material success. Gradually, David started reconnecting with old passions—writing, volunteering, and spending quality time with loved ones. These small acts of authenticity helped him begin to craft a new sense of purpose rooted in personal meaning rather than external validation.

David's story, while fictional, echoes the all-too-common theme of a *midlife crisis*: the moment when life's routines give way to introspection. It's a time when many face their mortality, question their choices, and grapple with the terror that life may lack inherent meaning. These feelings are uncomfortable but ultimately a vital part of living authentically.

His journey towards clarity illustrates that confronting his existential anxiety—acknowledging mortality, seeking personal purpose, and embracing freedom—can lead to renewal. The midlife crisis, in this light, becomes not just a crisis but an opportunity for rebirth—a chance to create a life aligned with one's deepest values and truths. It's a path many take, whether consciously or through circumstance, learning that even in facing uncertainty, we regain our capacity for meaning, love, and authentic existence.

Existential Therapy Concepts in Practice

As previously noted, existential therapists view *existential anxiety* as originating from four primary sources: freedom and responsibility, the need for meaning, the fundamental experience of being alone in the world, and awareness of death. Let's look at some simple, actionable techniques rooted in existentialist thought that you can use right now to help you live more authentically and find your own sense of purpose.

Reflect on What Truly Matters

Start by carving out time each week for reflection. Ask yourself: "What are the values that truly matter to me? What kind of life would I find meaningful?" Write down your thoughts. Many existentialists believe that life's meaning isn't something outside us but something we create ourselves. By clarifying your core values—whether kindness, creativity, connection, or growth—you establish a foundation to live intentionally.

For example, if honesty or compassion is important to you, consider how your daily actions align with those values. Are there ways to incorporate them more intentionally?

This exercise helps you craft a life that authentically reflects your inner priorities—an antidote to living on autopilot or merely reacting to external expectations.

Practice Mindfulness and Acceptance

Existentialist therapy often emphasizes embracing life's uncertainties rather than fighting them. Practice mindfulness—pay close attention to your thoughts, feelings, and sensations without judgment. When fears about death or meaning surface, instead of suppressing or denying them, observe them with curiosity.

For instance, if you notice a thought like "I'm going to fail," acknowledge it calmly, then explore what that fear signifies. Ask yourself: "What does failure mean to me? Can I accept that uncertainty is part of being human?" Accepting the limits of life can bring a surprising sense of peace. It's not about resignation but about courageously facing reality, which allows you to act authentically despite fears.

Use Thought Experiments to Clarify Your Existence

One powerful technique involves imagining scenarios where you confront your fears about mortality or insignificance. For example, picture yourself at the end of your life—what would you want to have accomplished? What relationships would you cherish? How would you want to be remembered?

This kind of visualization—what existentialists call *death awareness exercises*—can help you prioritize what truly matters. It's a way to turn the fear of death into motivation, encouraging you to live fully in the present and focus on what adds genuine value to your life.

Build Authenticity by Facing Your Fears

Existentialist therapy invites you to act authentically—aligned with your values—rather than avoiding uncomfortable truths. Start small: if you feel anxious about speaking your mind, practice expressing your opinions in safe settings. If isolation frightens you, seek opportunities to connect with others gradually, even if it's a brief conversation.

This process isn't about eliminating fear but learning to live alongside it. By intentionally engaging with what makes you uncomfortable in a controlled way, you strengthen your capacity to face life's inevitable uncertainties with courage. Think of it as lifting weights—you get stronger by confronting resistance, not avoiding it.

Find Meaning in Small Moments

Finally, remember that existentialism isn't about making grand gestures. It's found in everyday choices—small acts of kindness, honest conversations, or pursuing a hobby that sparks your passion. The philosopher Albert Camus suggested that we create meaning through rebellion against life's absurdity, and that rebellion can be as simple as choosing to live with integrity.

Each day, ask yourself: "What small act can I do today that aligns with my core values? How can I bring awareness and intention into my routine?" These little moments accumulate, helping you build a more authentic and meaningful life.

Journaling Prompts

1. What are the values or beliefs that give your life a sense of purpose? How do you live in accordance with them?

2. When faced with uncertainty or the unknown, how do you respond? Do you embrace it or try to avoid it?

3. In what ways do you feel in control of your life? Where do you feel helpless or overwhelmed?

4. How do you find meaning in everyday life? What small actions or routines bring you a sense of fulfillment?

5. What are the biggest fears or concerns you have about your life or mortality?

6. When you reflect on the idea that life might have no inherent meaning, and that we have to find it ourselves, how does that make you feel?

7. Are there situations or thoughts that trigger existential fears? How do you usually react?

8. Do you tend to deny or push aside thoughts about death and life's purpose? What happens when you do?

9. When faced with life's uncertainties, what thoughts or beliefs help you cope? Which ones increase your anxiety?

10. Can you relate to David's feelings of restlessness and questioning? How do you handle similar moments of doubt or fear?

11. Think about times when you've experienced a loss or significant change. How did those moments challenge your sense of purpose?

12. How do you think confronting mortality and uncertainty could change your approach to life?

13. What small daily actions can you take to reconnect with your core values and purpose?

14. When you have intrusive or anxious thoughts about mortality, what thoughts and perspectives can help you gently shift your focus?

15. What activities or rituals—such as reflection, gratitude, or meaningful connection—do you find helpful for confronting existential fears?

Journaling

Journaling

Chapter Eleven

Substance Abuse and Its Relationship With Anxiety

THE RELATIONSHIP BETWEEN ANXIETY and substance abuse has been so well documented, especially in some specific anxiety disorders, that I feel it would be a disservice to my readers if I didn't address the subject in this book. There are a number of reasons for this relationship, which we will discuss in this chapter. Most importantly, though, I approached this chapter with the thought of providing helpful advice and specific techniques that individuals can use to help deal with the issue of substance abuse. It should also be noted that substance abuse implies addiction, and also that substance abuse isn't the only kind of addiction that can manifest itself as a strategy for anxiety reduction.

Is Substance Abuse Really a Problem

According to an article from the NIH's website (National Institute for Health), 33 .38% of individuals who sought treatment for an alcohol use disorder also had at least one co-occurring independent anxiety disorder. NCS-R (National Comorbidity Survey Replication) data indicate that individuals with an anxiety disorder are more likely to develop a substance use disorder compared to those without an anxiety disorder. Around 35-40% of individuals with Generalized Anxiety Disorder (GAD) and approximately

20-30% of individuals with some kind of anxiety disorder report a co-existing substance use disorder at some point in their lifetime.

These statistics reinforce my own clinical experience. The clinic that I worked in for my internship saw a lot of clientele from the correctional system. Many of the felons that I worked with had some kind of substance abuse from their past. For some, that was how they had come to find themselves in the prison system to begin with. The vast majority of them had post traumatic stress from the prison system alone, but many also had some kind of traumatic experiences from the past. It's a very sad fact that many individuals with significant trauma struggle with alcohol use, particularly veterans of war. As you'll see, there are a variety of reasons for this. In my profession, we refer to this type of behavior as "self-medication." As you might infer from the phrase, we think that the substance is being used to suppress the symptoms of their anxiety disorder (in many cases, PTSD).

Substances of Choice for Self-Medicating Anxiety

Anxiety disorders and substance use disorders frequently overlap, a fact that often complicates the treatment of both conditions. Individuals experiencing anxiety symptoms may turn to various substances seeking relief, inadvertently creating a cycle of dependency. Understanding the substances of choice and their effects provides insight into this complex interaction, highlighting the necessity for nuanced treatment strategies.

Alcohol as a Social Lubricant and Sedative

Alcohol is one of the most commonly used substances for self-medication among individuals with anxiety disorders. Its sedative effects are appealing, especially for those struggling with symptoms like chronic worry, social anxiety, or panic attacks. Alcohol's depressant properties work by enhancing the effects of the neurotransmitter gamma-aminobutyric acid (GABA), which inhibits brain activity and produces calming effects.

Research indicates that individuals with social anxiety disorder, for example, might use alcohol to ease tension and facilitate social interactions, turning it into a so-called "social lubricant" (Cox et al., 1988). However, this temporary relief often comes at a cost. Chronic use can lead to dependency, exacerbation of anxiety symptoms during withdrawal, and impairments in cognitive and emotional functioning over time.

Prescription Medications: Benzodiazepines and Misuse

Benzodiazepines, such as diazepam (Valium) and alprazolam (Xanax), are frequently prescribed for acute anxiety management due to their rapid onset and effectiveness in reducing symptoms. They increase GABA activity, similar to alcohol, alleviating anxiety quickly. However, their potential for misuse is significant. Individuals may use these medications beyond prescribed limits to manage persistent anxiety symptoms, risking tolerance and dependence.

A study by Voshaar et al. (2006) examined the patterns of benzodiazepine misuse among patients with anxiety, highlighting cases where prescriptions continued long-term without adequate evaluation of ongoing necessity. The misuse arises from individuals seeking sustained relief, emphasizing these medications' role in perpetuating substance use issues if not carefully monitored.

Marijuana: Perceived Relief and Risks

With increasing legalization, marijuana is another substance sought for self-medication. Some users report it helps with anxiety, potentially due to its ability to alter the endocannabinoid system, which plays a role in stress and emotional regulation (Childs et al., 2017). Despite anecdotal evidence, the relationship is paradoxical. While low doses might reduce anxiety for some, high doses or chronic use can exacerbate anxiety symptoms, affect cognitive function, and lead to dependency.

In states where marijuana remains illegal, using it to alleviate anxiety brings significant legal risks. Possession and distribution can result in criminal charges, potentially leading to fines, imprisonment, or a permanent criminal record, impacting future employment and housing opportunities. Additionally, federal law still classifies marijuana as a Schedule I substance, complicating its legal status even in states where it's permitted for recreational or medical use. These legal discrepancies emphasize the importance of seeking alternative, lawful treatment methods for anxiety management, prioritizing mental health support through licensed professionals (Pacula et al., 2014).

The Danger of Self-Medication

While these substances may offer temporary relief for anxiety, they often lead to a vicious cycle of dependency, worsened symptoms, and reduced quality of life. Self-medication can mask underlying issues, delay proper treatment, and increase the risk of developing co-occurring disorders. Recognizing the substances used and their effects highlights the importance of a comprehensive treatment approach that simultaneously addresses anxiety and substance use.

Effective Treatment Models for Substance Use Disorders

Effective treatment approaches for individuals with Substance Use Disorders (SUDs) and anxiety disorders incorporate a variety of theoretical models that address the multifaceted nature of addiction. When effectively combined, these models offer a comprehensive approach toward recovery, addressing not just the symptoms of substance use but underlying causes and broader life implications. Keep in mind that these disorders are complex, influenced by numerous factors including genetic, environmental, and psychological components.

The Medical Model

The medical model treats SUDs primarily as chronic brain diseases, emphasizing the role of neurobiology in addiction. This model asserts that addiction is driven by changes in brain function caused by prolonged substance use, and thus requires medical intervention. Treatments often include pharmacological approaches, such as methadone for opioid use disorder or naltrexone for alcohol dependence, which help manage withdrawal symptoms and reduce cravings (Volkow et al., 2009).

The Psychological Models

Psychological models focus on the cognitive, emotional, and behavioral aspects of SUDs. Cognitive Behavioral Therapy (CBT) is one of the most commonly employed psychological models, aimed at changing maladaptive thought patterns that fuel substance use. Research shows CBT helps clients recognize and restructure thoughts, develop coping strategies, and improve problem-solving skills (Carroll, 1998).

Motivational Interviewing (MI), another effective psychological approach, enhances clients' intrinsic motivation to change by resolving ambivalence and promoting a commitment to recovery. MI's empathetic, client-centered style has been particularly effective in engaging clients' resistant to change (Miller & Rollnick, 2002).

The Biopsychosocial Model

This is an integrative model that recognizes SUDs stem from a combination of biological, psychological, and social factors. It advocates for holistic treatment plans tailored to individuals' comprehensive needs, addressing not just physical addiction, but psychological health and social environments as well. Interventions might include family therapy, individual counseling, and social support systems, ensuring recovery is sustainable beyond treatment (Engel, 1977).

The Social Models

Social models posit that addiction is greatly influenced by one's environment, social networks, and community. One prominent example is the 12-Step Model, famously used by Alcoholics Anonymous (AA) and Narcotics Anonymous (NA). These programs highlight the importance of community support, encouraging members to work through the 12 steps of recovery and emphasizing spirituality, peer support, and personal accountability. Studies consistently find that participation in 12-step programs can significantly enhance outcomes when combined with traditional treatment (Ouimette et al., 1998).

Practical Techniques You Can Use

Although we've discussed many practical techniques for individual use with anxiety management in past chapters, let's review and expand on them.

Developing Mindfulness and Grounding Techniques

Mindfulness-based practices are increasingly recognized as effective tools for reducing anxiety and facilitating sobriety. Regular mindfulness exercises, such as deep breathing, body scans, or focused attention on sensory experiences, help individuals stay present and reduce rumination—the internal chatter that fuels anxiety. A study by Hofmann, Sawyer, Witt, and Oh (2010) demonstrates that mindfulness-based interventions significantly decrease anxiety symptoms. For individuals with substance use issues, mindfulness also enhances awareness of cravings and urges, making it easier to resist acting on impulses to use substances as a form of self-medication (Garland, 2013). Practicing mindfulness daily builds tolerance for uncomfortable feelings and promotes healthier emotional regulation.

If that's too abstract for you, let's look at what an example of what one of these types of exercises looks like: *Find a quiet space and sit comfortably, either in a chair or on the floor, allowing your hands to rest naturally. Close your eyes and take three deep breaths, focusing on your abdomen expanding and contracting. As thoughts and feelings arise, acknowledge each one without judgment, labeling them as "thinking" or "feeling." Visualize each thought or feeling as a leaf floating down a stream, letting them drift away naturally. Accept their presence without needing to change or act on them, repeating the mantra: "I notice you, and it's OK for you to be here." Refocus on your breathing, letting the rhythmic rise and fall anchor you in the present moment. Gradually bring your awareness back to your surroundings, reflecting on any changes in your mood or perspective. Carry this mindfulness with you throughout the day, using it as a tool to manage anxiety and remain present.*

Keep in mind that there are many YouTube videos that you can use as a tutorial for mindfulness and meditation practices. Additionally, there are mindfulness and meditation apps that you can download on various devices, such as cellphones, laptops, and tablets.

Cognitive Behavioral Strategies for Challenging Negative Thought Patterns

Many individuals with anxiety and substance dependence are caught in a cycle of negative thinking—believing that they cannot cope without substances or that their anxiety will inevitably overwhelm them. Cognitive Behavioral Therapy (CBT) techniques can help break this cycle. For example, someone might journal about their automatic thoughts, such as "I won't survive this panic attack," and then systematically challenge and reframe these beliefs. By identifying cognitive distortions—like catastrophizing or overgeneralization—and replacing them with realistic, compassionate thoughts, individuals weaken the emotional grip of anxiety and reduce the fear of withdrawal or relapse (Beck, 1976). These internal shifts increase confidence to face anxiety-provoking situations without resorting to substances.

Establishing a Routine and Structured Environment

Unpredictability and chaos can intensify both anxiety and substance cravings. Establishing a daily routine—including fixed times for meals, exercise, relaxation, and sleep—creates a sense of safety and control. Research by Tuithof et al. (2017) indicates that stability and predictability are protective factors that reduce relapse in substance users. Structured environments help individuals manage anxiety by reducing uncertainty and offer clear pathways for handling distress without resorting to impulsive substance use.

Seeking Social Support and Accountability

Isolation often worsens both anxiety and substance dependence. Building a support network—whether through trusted friends, family members, support groups, or mental health professionals—provides emotional validation and practical accountability. Group therapies like Alcoholics Anonymous (AA) or SMART Recovery connect individuals facing similar struggles, reducing feelings of loneliness and shame (Kelly, 2017). Regular interaction within these groups fosters social skills, reassurance, and shared hope, helping individuals stay committed to their recovery and manage anxiety more effectively.

Implementing Urge Surfing and Craving Management Techniques

Cravings and urges, particularly during anxiety spikes, can feel overwhelming. Techniques like urge surfing teach individuals to observe and accept cravings without acting on them. Rather than trying to suppress a craving, the person notes the sensation, observes it as temporary, and allows it to rise and fall like a wave. This process, supported by mindfulness practices, reduces the likelihood of relapse triggered by cravings (Davidson et al., 2009). Recognizing that these urges are transient helps individuals develop patience and resilience.

Urge surfing involves observing cravings non-judgmentally rather than acting on them, allowing them to crest and subside naturally like waves. Begin by finding a quiet space and acknowledging the urge without labeling it as good or bad. Focus on physical sensations associated with the craving, like tightness or warmth, identifying where you feel them in your body. Visualize the craving as a wave, noticing how it intensifies, peaks, and eventually dissipates. Practice deep breathing, focusing on each breath as you "ride" the wave of the craving. Remind yourself that urges are temporary and that you have the strength to let them pass without succumbing. With regular practice, urge surfing can increase your tolerance for discomfort and reduce the power cravings hold over you, fostering healthier self-control and resilience.

Addressing Underlying Trauma and Past Experiences

Substances are often used to cope with unresolved trauma or adverse childhood experiences that fuel anxiety. Trauma-focused therapies—such as Eye Movement Desensitization and Reprocessing (EMDR) or trauma-informed CBT—can help process these experiences, reducing their power to trigger substance use as a coping mechanism. Healing emotional wounds diminishes one of the root causes of both anxiety and addiction, fostering healthier emotional regulation (Kezelman & Stavropoulos, 2012).

Trauma-focused imagery reprocessing involves guiding an individual to safely revisit and reframe traumatic memories, reducing their emotional impact over time. For this, a person begins by thinking about the traumatic event in a controlled, guided way—focusing on details, sensations, and thoughts—while practicing relaxation techniques like deep breathing to stay calm. As you become more comfortable, you work to reinterpret the memory, shifting from feelings of helplessness or shame to understanding and empowerment. For example, you might visualize yourself confronting and overcoming the trauma, perhaps a bully or abusive parent, instilling a sense of confidence in yourself and role-playing how you might deal with similar scenarios in the future. Practicing this regularly can lessen intrusive thoughts and emotional distress associated with past trauma. By integrating this technique into daily routines, you can gradually lessen the hold of traumatic memories, fostering a sense of safety and control, rebuilding your emotional strength.

Medication as an Adjunct When Needed

For some individuals, medication can be a helpful adjunct to therapy by reducing the intensity of anxiety symptoms, cravings, and withdrawal effects. Selective serotonin reuptake inhibitors (SSRIs), such as sertraline and escitalopram, are commonly prescribed and have been shown to decrease generalized anxiety and improve mood, which may lessen the urge to self-medicate (Bandelow & Michaelis, 2015). Benzodiazepines can provide immediate relief but are recommended only for short-term use due to the risk of dependency. The key is combining medication under supervision with behavioral therapies to address both the physiological and psychological facets of anxiety and substance dependence.

Building Long-term Resilience Through Meaning and Purpose

Finally, engaging in activities that foster a sense of meaning can provide a resilient foundation. Viktor Frankl's logotherapy emphasizes the importance of discovering purpose, such as volunteering, pursuing hobbies, or connecting deeply with loved ones. When individuals find intrinsic value in life beyond substance use, their motivation to maintain sobriety and manage anxiety increases. Journaling, expression through arts, or spiritual practices can help cultivate this sense of purpose, serving as a protective buffer against relapse.

Case Study: Jason's Dual Battle — Managing Anxiety and Substance Dependence

Jason is a 32-year-old man living in a bustling city. Until recently, he seemed to balance his life reasonably well—working in a marketing firm, maintaining friendships, and engaging in hobbies. However, over the past three years, Jason's life grew increasingly chaotic. What started as occasional alcohol use to unwind after stressful days turned into a daily habit, and soon, he found himself relying heavily on alcohol and prescription pills to cope with relentless anxiety.

Jason's anxiety symptoms began subtly: racing thoughts, stomachaches, and difficulty sleeping. But as work pressures mounted and personal relationships became strained, his anxiety intensified. During especially stressful periods—such as layoffs or relationship crises—Jason would binge drink or misuse prescription medications to numb the overwhelming feelings. Sometimes, he drank or took pills just to calm his mind enough to get through each day, fearing if he didn't, his anxiety might spiral out of control altogether.

His dependency on substances took a toll, affecting his health, work performance, and relationships. His friends noticed he was becoming more withdrawn, and he frequently canceled plans, claiming exhaustion or stress. Jason himself felt trapped—he wanted to stop abusing substances but couldn't face the anxiety without their numbing effect. This vicious cycle deepened, leading to feelings of shame and hopelessness.

Eventually, Jason realized he needed help. After a particularly bad episode where he drank heavily and felt an intense panic attack, he reached out to a mental health professional. During his first appointment, he described his struggles with persistent anxiety, substance dependency, and the destructive cycle they fueled. The clinician conducted a comprehensive assessment, recognizing that Jason was dealing with both an anxiety disorder and substance use disorder, which complicate each other.

The therapist explained that Jason's symptoms fit with Generalized Anxiety Disorder and Substance Use Disorder, requiring an integrated treatment approach. Together, they designed a plan to manage both issues simultaneously. The initial focus was on stabilizing his mood and reducing substance intake, while building skills to confront his anxiety without relying on alcohol and pills.

Jason was introduced to Cognitive Behavioral Therapy (CBT), which helped him identify negative thought patterns contributing to his anxiety, such as "I can't handle stress without substances" or "I'll fail if I try to change." Through exercises, he learned to challenge these beliefs, replacing catastrophic thoughts with more realistic ones like, "I can cope with stress in healthier ways" or "I've managed difficult times before; I can do it again."

A core part of his therapy involved gradual exposure to anxiety-provoking situations. Starting with small steps—such as practicing mindfulness or relaxation techniques during stressful moments—Jason gradually worked toward facing larger fears, like speaking up in meetings or attending social events, without turning to substances. His therapist also worked with him on developing healthier coping skills, including deep breathing, progressive muscle relaxation, and engaging in hobbies like running or drawing to reduce his anxiety naturally.

In addition to therapy, Jason engaged in a medically supervised detox program to safely reduce his substance dependence. He also received support for managing cravings and recognizing triggers that prompted substance use—like specific stressful events or feelings of loneliness. Regular check-ins with a psychiatrist helped monitor his medication, which included an SSRI to balance his anxiety symptoms, along with support to prevent relapse.

Over the following months, Jason began to notice subtle but significant improvements. His anxiety episodes became less frequent and intense, and he found himself able to manage stress more effectively using the skills learned in therapy. His dependency on alcohol and pills decreased steadily; he used his coping strategies instead of substances during stressful events. Jason started reconnecting with friends and re-engaging with activities he loved, feeling a renewed sense of control over his life.

High Stress Work and Substance Abuse

If you can relate to the story of Jason, you are not alone. High stress jobs that require a person to perform at a peak level of professionalism on a consistent basis are well known to be breeding grounds for substance abusers. Some examples of such jobs might include professional sports athletes, performing musicians, surgeons, actors, fighter pilots, CEOs, police officers, and other first responders. Obviously, that doesn't mean that you should conclude that workers in such fields are all substance abusers. I just mean that these fields can be very highly stressful for the people working in them.

You often hear of actors and musicians speaking out about their struggles with substance abuse. I don't really want to list off a bunch of names, because I don't like to spend too much time talking about specific individuals and their real life struggles. I will, however, mention Matthew Perry and his struggles with substance abuse, as he was very open about the subject. It's so common to hear about entertainers struggling with anxiety and substance abuse that it's almost cliché at this point. If you don't know who Matthew Perry is, I will give a very brief summary.

Matthew Perry, best known for his role as Chandler Bing on the hit television show *Friends*, has openly shared his battles with anxiety and substance abuse. At the height of his fame in the 1990s, Perry faced intense pressure and scrutiny, which aggravated his underlying anxiety. To cope, he turned to prescription painkillers and alcohol, leading to a severe cycle of addiction that often overshadowed his professional success. Despite several publicized struggles with sobriety, Perry's journey embodies resilience. He actively sought treatment through rehabilitation programs and used his platform to raise awareness about addiction and mental health, advocating for recovery and offering hope to those facing similar challenges. Perry's transparency about his struggles highlighted his ongoing battle between anxiety and substance dependence, showcasing the importance of seeking help and embracing vulnerability.

Although Matthew Perry tragically passed away in 2023, his story is important. His story highlights the fact that success can bring its own difficulties and challenges. It also highlights the fact that, with consistent effort, you can overcome even a very serious substance abuse problem. That has implications for all of us. I use examples of celebrities, public figures, and historical figures who struggle with problems so that you know that even the most successful people in the world struggle with psychological problems. You aren't alone.

Journaling Prompts

1. Was there ever a time when you turned to a substance to cope with anxiety? What was the immediate effect, and how did you feel afterward?

2. Identify your go-to behaviors when feeling stressed or anxious. How do you think these choices impact your well-being and anxiety levels in the long run?

3. Are there any situations that trigger your desire to self-medicate with substances? What emotions or thoughts accompany these moments?

4. What beliefs do you hold about using substances to manage anxiety or stress? How might questioning these beliefs change your actions?

5. Write about patterns you notice in your anxiety coping behaviors. Are there any situations where you are more likely to rely on substances?

6. Think about a recent moment of anxiety or craving. How might using cognitive-behavioral strategies have altered your response?

7. Reflect on a time when you successfully used an alternative coping skill instead of substances. What made it effective for you?

8. If you struggle with substance abuse, how might creating a structured daily routine help reduce your anxiety and substance use tendencies? Describe your ideal routine.

9. Consider your support network. How can reaching out to friends, family, or support groups improve your management of anxiety?

10. Visualize implementing "urge surfing" the next time you experience a craving. What do you notice as you ride the wave of the craving?

11. Consider Jason's journey from the case study. In what ways do you relate to his experiences with anxiety and substance use?

12. How might Jason's use of CBT techniques inspire changes in how you manage anxiety and substance use (if you are using)?

13. Reflect on the turning point when Jason sought help. What would seeking help look like for you, and what support do you envision on your journey?

14. In what ways do Jason's coping skills resonate with you? How can they inspire you to explore new strategies?

15. Write about any insights gained from recognizing cycles of anxiety and substance use in Jason's story. How can these insights guide your path to healing?

Journaling

Journaling

Chapter Twelve

Sticking Points, Final Thoughts

As we come to the final chapter, I want to leave you with an important component of the process that you began from the moment you bought this book: what to do when we hit sticking points and road blocks on the path to a better life. One of the things that really motivated me to write a chapter like this was the realization that I came to one day while working with a client. He seemed to have worked out exactly what he needed to do during our previous session, yet hadn't reported taking any meaningful action since that session. We talked about why he couldn't seem to take the next step. We might have even talked about it in another later session. What was going on here, I wondered. Sure, you might chalk it up to the client just being lazy, or indecisive. But I kept running into this scenario with several of my other clients. They would come to a point where they needed to take action to move ahead in their lives, and then... nothing. Why? Well, the answer might not be as simple as we would like, but researchers have discovered and studied this phenomenon before, in some detail. So, although answers in the field of psychology are never completely clear, at least we can have some level of insight into the process of change.

To set the stage for this section, I'd like to open with an introduction to James Prochaska's work, known as the "Transtheoretical Model of Behavior Change." This may sound strange or overly technical, but it just means that it incorporates ideas and concepts from several different theoretical models of psychotherapy. The model is meant to help us understand the different stages of change that people move through in their lives so that we can understand that every individual may need something different to move them forward in their process of change, depending on what stage they are at in the process.

Prochaska's Transtheoretical Model of Behavior Change

The Transtheoretical Model of Behavior Change (TTM), introduced by James Prochaska and colleagues, is often applied to health-related behaviors like quitting smoking, adopting exercise routines, or achieving weight loss, but the model's principles can be applied to a diverse range of personal changes. Central to the TTM is the understanding that change is a process, not an event, and encompasses five key stages.

Stage One: Precontemplation

In the precontemplation stage, individuals are not yet considering change. They may be unaware that their behavior is problematic or see their behavior as something beyond control. Those in this stage often underestimate the benefits of change and emphasize the costs, fostering reluctance or resistance to change. For instance, a smoker might rationalize smoking as a stress reliever without considering the long-term health risks. Key characteristics of this stage include: lack of awareness about the need for change; low motivation or perceived self-efficacy (belief in one's likelihood to succeed); reliance on denial or defensiveness.

Progress from precontemplation can begin when individuals receive new information or experiences that confront their denial, raising awareness. Effective strategies to move forward include education, validation of feelings, and encouragement to think critically about one's habits.

Stage Two: Contemplation

During the contemplation stage, individuals acknowledge the possibility of change and begin considering it, albeit ambivalently. They weigh the pros and cons and assess potential benefits and barriers. Although they recognize their habits are problematic, they may linger in this stage for long periods without taking action, a process known as "chronic contemplation" or "behavioral procrastination." Key characteristics of this stage include: increased awareness of pros and cons; ambivalence about change; planning to take action in the foreseeable future, typically within six months. As you've been reading this book, you may find yourself in the contemplation stage, trying to decide what you need to do, what steps you need to take to move forward and resolve your anxiety.

For this stage, progress involves strengthening self-efficacy and self-motivation, as you strive to resolve your ambivalence. Motivational interviewing, exploring personal values, and addressing perceived barriers can be beneficial in this stage. Motivational interviewing usually involves working with some kind of professional helper: a psychologist, counselor, or other. It involves exploring your reasons for wanting change and your concerns about maintaining the status quo. This professional would help you reduce your ambivalence as you resolve conflicting thoughts and feelings about change. They would help foster your internal motivation to make positive changes. Additionally, your helper would work towards establishing a sense of belief in your ability to achieve your goals. Finally, the helper would work with you to develop a specific and achievable plan of action as you begin to move forward.

Stage Three: Preparation

Perhaps, as you have been reading this book, you have entered the preparation phase. The preparation stage is marked by commitment to change and planning actionable steps. Individuals in this stage have decided to change and are preparing to initiate action. They might experiment with small changes, such as cutting down on cigarette consumption or researching workout plans. This stage often includes setting specific goals and gathering resources or support, like joining a cessation group or finding an accountability partner.

The key characteristics of this stage are: intention to take immediate action, usually within the next month; an increasing belief in the ability to change (self-efficacy); the development of a concrete and realistic action plan. Progressing from preparation may require support to design and implement a feasible action plan. It's important to seek encouragement as you begin planning achievable goals.

Stage Four: Action

In the action stage, individuals actively implement their change strategies, committing significant time and energy to modify their behaviors. This stage is where change is most visible—people might stop smoking completely, start a regular exercise routine, or adopt a healthier diet. Success in this stage involves consistently practicing new habits and replacing old behaviors, a process that requires strong willpower and resistance to temptation. If you have already taken meaningful action based on the concepts presented in earlier chapters, congratulations! That means that you are in the action stage, or have moved through it, and that is actually very impressive!

The key characteristics for the action phase are: implementation of behavior change strategies; active adjustment of environment and social support to sustain change; and high risk for relapse, necessitating coping strategies. Navigating this stage effectively involves: recognizing triggers, using positive reinforcement, seeking continuous support, and celebrating progress to bolster confidence and sustain momentum. Building routines and practicing stress management are crucial for avoiding a relapse into old, familiar patterns of behavior.

Stage Five: Maintenance

The maintenance stage continues from the action stage, sustaining new behavior over the long term by preventing relapse and consolidating gains made during the action phase. The risk of returning to old habits decreases, but vigilance and deliberate effort continue to be necessary. Individuals in this stage assimilate their new behaviors into their lifestyle and identity, finding satisfaction and stability in their achievements.

For stage five, key characteristic are: ongoing evaluation and adjustment of strategies to sustain change; increased self-confidence in maintaining new behavior; and development of a supportive environment that reinforces change. Strategies for sustained change involve continued self-monitoring, long-term goal setting, maintaining motivation through positive reminders, and engaging in community or peer support networks. Recognizing potential stressors and devising proactive countermeasures help prevent setbacks.

Common Challenges to Making Lifestyle Changes

As you continue on your path to wellness, you may find that you have to make lifestyle changes. Maybe the anxiety type that you're dealing with is best dealt with through a lifestyle change. Or maybe you need to practice doing CBT worksheets to think through your anxious thoughts in a more logical manner. And even if your anxiety type is best treated with medications, you probably don't want to be on those medications forever. That means you will probably need to begin making some lifestyle changes. We've already talked about the Transtheoretical Model (TTM), but now I want to discuss some other potential impediments to moving forward, and how we can overcome them.

The Comfort of Familiarity: A Psychological Barrier to Change

One of the most significant psychological barriers to implementing change in one's life is the powerful draw of familiarity. The comfort of familiarity refers to the human preference for the known and predictable, even when it comes at the cost of foregoing potential benefits that change could bring. This innate preference for routine and existing patterns is deeply rooted in our psychology, often operating below conscious awareness as a mechanism for maintaining psychological stability.

Familiarity is soothing because it reduces uncertainty, a state that naturally provokes anxiety and distress. When individuals are faced with the prospect of change, the mere idea of moving away from what is known can trigger subconscious resistance. This resistance is often not a rejection of change itself but rather an aversion to the potential discomfort that accompanies transitioning to something new.

The theory of "cognitive consonance," as coined in psychological literature, suggests that people strive for harmony within their beliefs, attitudes, and behaviors. Familiar routines provide a sense of consonance, making life feel orderly and manageable. Conversely, change introduces cognitive dissonance, a state of mental tension that arises when new behaviors threaten established beliefs or routines, prompting individuals to cling tightly to the familiar.

Additionally, change requires not only an adaptation to new behaviors but also a dismantling of long-standing habits and cognitive schemas. This dismantling process is endowed with emotional attachments accrued over time. Thus, the sense of loss associated with leaving behind the familiarity of existing habits can be a daunting challenge to overcome.

In essence, the comfort of familiarity acts as a protective buffer against the chaos and unpredictability of the external world, creating an invisible yet powerful barrier to change. Overcoming this barrier involves consciously recognizing the allure of familiarity and embracing the discomfort of change as an opportunity for growth, driven by a commitment to personal development and resiliency.

Behavioral Patterns and Habits

When embarking on the journey of personal change, one of the most formidable challenges individuals encounter is breaking free from established behavioral patterns and habits. Habits are powerful because they are ingrained responses that operate largely outside of conscious awareness, cultivated through repetition until they become automatic.

At the core of habit formation is the habit loop, a psychological pattern first described by researchers like Charles Duhigg in "The Power of Habit." This loop consists of a cue, which triggers the behavior (the routine or behavior itself) and the reward that reinforces it. Over time, this loop becomes a neural pathway in the brain, making the habit increasingly automatic and difficult to disrupt.

Changing habits requires not only identifying the cues and rewards that sustain them but also implementing consistent alternative behaviors. This is challenging because habits, by nature, resist change. They are the brain's way of conserving energy, allowing us to perform tasks without expending excessive mental effort. When an individual attempts to change a long-standing habit, the brain instinctively resists, prioritizing efficiency over change.

The key to overcoming entrenched behavioral patterns lies in consistency. However, maintaining consistency can prove challenging due to the tendency to revert to familiar routines, especially in times of stress. This is compounded by the often tedious process of developing new habits, which requires repeated, deliberate practice before becoming automatic.

Another complicating factor is the context in which habits occur. Environmental cues—from the sights and sounds around us to social settings and times of day—can powerfully influence our behaviors. Successfully changing a habit often necessitates altering or managing these cues, which can be inconvenient or impractical for some individuals.

Effectively changing behavioral patterns involves a multifaceted approach. Setting clear, attainable goals that align with personal values provides motivation and direction. Breaking down the desired change into smaller, manageable steps ensures gradual progress, minimizing feelings of being overwhelmed. Employing habit-reversal techniques, such as substituting a new, healthier behavior for the old one, can be highly effective. Additionally, using reinforcement strategies to reward new habit formations encourages sustained commitment, so make sure to reward yourself early and often as you begin substituting your new behavior. Lastly, involving a support system—friends, family, or professional coaches—provides accountability and encouragement, which are critical for long-term success.

While challenging, altering behavioral patterns and habits is entirely achievable through consistent effort, strategic planning, and the leveraging of supportive networks. Recognizing the complexity and providing patience and diligence can help individuals transcend habitual barriers, leading to meaningful and lasting change.

Motivational Challenges

Motivational challenges are a common obstacle in the journey of implementing lifestyle changes. At the start, there is often a surge of motivation—an inner desire to improve or evolve—that propels individuals forward. However, as time progresses, maintaining that motivation can become difficult, especially when faced with setbacks, fatigue, or slower progress than expected. This decline in enthusiasm can lead to decreased effort and even abandonment of goals altogether. A significant factor influencing motivation is whether the drive is intrinsic or extrinsic. Intrinsic motivation, which comes from personal satisfaction and the inherent joy of the activity, tends to be more sustainable over the long term because it aligns with an individual's values and sense of purpose. Conversely, extrinsic motivation—driven by external rewards like weight loss, approval, or societal pressures—may provide short-term motivation but often lacks the depth required for lasting change.

Another challenge arises from setting vague or unrealistic goals. When goals are broad or undefined, such as simply wanting to "get healthier," it becomes hard to measure progress or experience a sense of achievement. This lack of clarity can dampen motivation, as there are fewer tangible milestones to celebrate. Emotions also significantly impact motivation—feelings of stress, anxiety, or low mood can sap energy and enthusiasm, making it harder to stay committed. When people are overwhelmed by negative emotions, they may doubt their ability to succeed or fear failure, which creates additional resistance to change.

Despite these challenges, certain strategies can help sustain motivation. Setting clear, specific, and achievable goals—often called SMART goals (Specific, Measurable, Achievable, Relevant, Time-bound)—can provide the structure needed for steady progress. Connecting those goals to personal values makes the process more meaningful, boosting intrinsic motivation. Visualization techniques, where one imagines successful outcomes and the positive feelings associated with them, can reinforce motivation during difficult times. Additionally, building accountability through support groups, friends, or mentors can encourage persistence by providing encouragement, feedback, and a sense of shared purpose. Overall, understanding these motivational hurdles and actively addressing them—by clarifying goals, aligning with personal values, visualizing success, and seeking social support—can help maintain enthusiasm and perseverance throughout the process of change.

Social and Environmental Influences

When trying to adopt new habits or make significant life changes, social and environmental influences can act as powerful barriers. These factors often shape our behaviors and attitudes in ways we may not fully realize, making change more difficult to sustain.

Social influences include the opinions, expectations, and behaviors of family, friends, and peers. For instance, if a person tries to quit smoking but their social circle continues to smoke or celebrates their continued use, it can create pressure to revert to old habits. Peer pressure can subtly—or overtly—encourage behaviors that contradict personal change goals. Additionally, societal norms and cultural practices can reinforce existing habits, making it harder to deviate from the status quo.

Environmental factors also play a significant role. The physical settings where we spend our time can either support or hinder behavior change. For example, someone trying to eat healthier may find it challenging if they live near convenience stores stocked with junk food, or if their workplace lacks healthy meal options. Similarly, if a person aims to exercise regularly but has no safe or accessible places to walk or workout, their motivation can decrease significantly.

Stressful or unstructured environments often make change more difficult, too. For example, chaotic home situations or stressful jobs can drain mental energy, making it harder to focus on long-term goals like quitting alcohol or improving mental health. In addition, environmental cues—like seeing others smoke or drink—can trigger cravings or temptations, especially if the environment is saturated with reminders of old habits.

Overcoming these challenges requires intentional effort. Creating a supportive environment involves re-designing daily routines to reduce exposure to triggers—such as replacing a smoking area with a designated stress-relief zone or stocking healthy foods at home. Socially, cultivating a supportive network of friends, family, or support groups who encourage rather than undermine your goals is vital. Sometimes, it also involves assertively communicating your needs and boundaries to those around you, so they understand and respect your journey. Recognizing the power of social and environmental influences is the first step toward reducing their impact, empowering you to create an internal and external landscape conducive to lasting change.

Cognitive Barriers

Our thoughts and beliefs play a crucial role in shaping how we approach change. When these cognitive patterns are negative or distorted, they can act as significant barriers, making it feel almost impossible to move forward. These mental blocks often operate beneath our awareness, subtly guiding our behaviors and reinforcing feelings of doubt, helplessness, or worthlessness.

One common cognitive barrier is *low self-efficacy*—the belief that we are incapable of successfully making or maintaining change. For example, someone trying to quit smoking might think, "I've failed before, so I won't succeed this time," which diminishes their motivation and increases the likelihood of giving up. This mindset creates a self-fulfilling prophecy where feelings of helplessness prevent action, reinforcing the cycle of inaction.

Another cognitive hurdle is *cognitive dissonance*—the mental discomfort that arises when our actions conflict with our beliefs or values. For instance, a person who values health but struggles with overeating might experience internal conflict, leading to feelings of guilt or shame. This discomfort can prompt justifications or denial, allowing the behavior to persist rather than confront the underlying issue.

Catastrophizing is yet another common cognitive distortion. When faced with the prospect of change, some individuals imagine the worst-case scenario—failing so miserably that it would ruin their lives. For example, someone may fear that giving up alcohol will lead to complete social breakdown or loss of all joy, thereby avoiding the effort altogether. These exaggerated fears block progress by magnifying temporary setbacks into insurmountable crises.

Overcoming these cognitive barriers involves actively challenging irrational or unhelpful thoughts. Techniques such as cognitive restructuring—examining evidence for and against negative beliefs—help to develop a more balanced outlook. Building awareness of automatic thoughts and replacing them with realistic statements fosters a sense of competence and hope. Additionally, developing internal dialogue that emphasizes progress and self-compassion can gradually diminish the power of these barriers, making change feel more attainable and less threatening. Recognizing and addressing negative thinking patterns allow us to clear mental obstacles and move confidently toward our goals.

Final Thoughts

Let's review some of the most important concepts that we've covered so far, starting with some of the basic concepts. Nearly everyone experiences some form of stress in their lives, at some point. This is the body's natural way of balancing the mental and physical resources with what we're facing. When we are experiencing challenges or in dangerous situations, our anxiety is activated. The important thing to remember is that normal anxiety is an adaptive, functional mechanism that is serving you. While it may seem tempting to want to eliminate all of our anxiety, we need it, just like any other emotion. The key is to resolve our anxiety, not banish it.

Most of us wrestle with some degree of anxiety just about every day of our lives: paying the bills, relationship stress, performance at work, getting homework done on time, global politics... the list goes on. Life is a balancing act, and we try to do our best to resolve the things in our lives that we feel anxious about. I call these things "every day stress," because we are confronted with these types of stressors on a regular basis. For most people, we are able to resolve these issues in our lives as they come up, and the anxiety clears up as we resolve them. However, for some people, the anxiety never seems to go away, no matter if they solve the problem or not. These people are displaying what psychologists call, "hypervigilance." Their brain is always on high alert, which is a symptom of Generalized Anxiety Disorder and also PTSD. People with these anxiety types may need a combination of medication and/or psychotherapy to help calm their nervous systems.

We've also discussed people who seem to have very specific fears and anxiety that often disrupt their every day life. These extremely specific fears and extreme anxiety responses often seem overly exaggerated to the majority of people in their lives. In some cases, these phobias can be eased by working through some of the worksheets that I provided in chapter 2, as it relates to risk management. Sometimes we need to rationally analyze just how much of a threat the actual phobia is to us, so that we can then assign an appropriate level of threat response to it. Yes, you could be in an elevator accident and it could result in your death. But most people could live 100,000 lifetimes worth of elevator trips and never experience a life threatening emergency in one. The same is true of flying and other forms of transportation. Sure, anything is possible, but if it is an extremely low probability event, then we should treat it as such. Having said that, a very common form of therapy with individuals with phobias is *exposure therapy*, because for most people with a phobia, the issue is that they have become hyper-sensitized to something. So, we expose people to smaller and less intimidating doses of their phobia, gradually working them up to the point where they can face their phobia head on.

Social interactions and performing in front of others is enough to terrify anyone. But people with Social Anxiety Disorder take this type of anxiety to a whole new level. These individuals often experience intense symptoms, such as a rapid heartbeat, trembling, and sweating. They can also have cognitive symptoms such as excessive self-consciousness and intense worry. Fortunately, a number of therapeutic interventions can be helpful for these individuals, including: CBT cognitive reframing, exposure therapy, breathing exercises, and (if necessary) anti-anxiety medication.

Everyone can probably relate to a time in their life when they felt frightened to the point of panic. Or perhaps you've had a series of events that came together over time that slowly built from feeling a little anxious to full on panic. In any case, we can all relate to the sensation of panic, but most of us don't have a chronic condition that seems to come and go at unpredictable times, with the degree of severity so intense that it can even feel like we're dying. That's what life is sometimes like for people with the anxiety type known as *panic disorder*. Fortunately, for these individuals, there are ways to regain a sense of control over life and minimize or even eliminate the panic attacks altogether. Therapy interventions such as CBT's reframing, medication, and lifestyle modifications (e.g. exercise and a balanced diet) can significantly mitigate the effects of the condition and help manage the symptoms when a panic attack does occur.

If you've ever dealt with anxiety surrounding fear of your partner cheating, fear of rejection or ghosting, feelings of anxiety whenever you and your partner are apart, and constant fixation on your relationship, then you can relate to individuals who struggle with *anxious attachment*. This type of anxiety is born of relationship dynamics that were at play during childhood. Psychologists call this failure to ultimately feel confident in the responsiveness of their caregivers *insecure attachment*. Fortunately, there are some things that help a lot with this type of anxiety. Firstly, just raising your awareness is helpful, as you can spot your emotional triggers and interpret those feelings in the context of your larger life experiences. Also, as usual, CBT is helpful with reframing your thoughts and beliefs about what is happening in your relationship so that you can keep your anxiety under control. Lifestyle changes such as exercise, combined with journaling and deep breathing exercises can provide effective coping mechanisms. Communicating your needs assertively, as well as setting healthy boundaries, will also generally help to keep relationships stable over time.

Existential anxiety is an anxiety type that just about every human being has experienced and can relate to. You might say that the root of existential anxiety comes from the universal fear that we humans seem to have of death and decay. This is likely why we detest living an inauthentic life so much, since we know that life is short and that we don't want to waste it living a lie. Existentialist philosophers and psychologists talked a lot about the importance of finding meaning in our lives and having our values aligned with our actions. I spoke about the cultural concept of the "midlife crisis" in chapter ten, pointing out that the drive for building a legacy with our lives is likely related to the pressure that existential anxiety places on us to leave something permanent behind after we are gone, to live beyond our own lifespan. The simple way to address this type of anxiety is to do the soul-searching necessary to answer the types of questions that existential anxiety poses to us: are you living an authentic life, are you chasing a life of meaning and purpose, what traces of your life will remain in the world long after you are gone? If you can come to the point of asking those questions, finding suitable answers to them, and having the courage to live them out in your life, you will most likely resolve your existential anxiety.

Throughout this book, we have touched on the subject of Cognitive Behavior Therapy, its techniques and benefits. CBT helps us by providing tools to question our beliefs by asking questions and challenging thought patterns such as *future prediction, mind reading,* and *discounting the positive,* among others. It's also helpful to spot when we're going on a downward emotional thought spiral. Be sure to make use of the cost/ benefit worksheet from chapter two if you feel like your anxious thoughts might be holding you back, and if you struggle with phobias, you might want to make use of the risk analysis worksheet to get a more realistic assessment of the risks that your phobia poses to you. Remember, the rational, logical mind that you have as a human is a massive asset to you when it comes to your mental health.

I want to leave you with some thoughts about medication from a clinician's perspective. Some people are completely anti-medication and, although I disagree with those people, I don't think that they should be forced to take medications against their will (unless they are obviously not of a sound mind). For some people that are suffering with extreme levels of anxiety, they can most likely benefit from short-term medication (or medications) that are set at an appropriate dosage by a professional. There are, of course, some risks that come with anti-anxiety medication. Namely, the risk of addiction and of relying completely on the medications as a crutch, rather than doing the work necessary to learn how to appropriately resolve and manage anxiety. This is why the general approach to medication should be: medication only as long as absolutely necessary, and only if the level of anxiety is so severe that it is disrupting the person's life to a degree that makes a normal life impossible. That means that the client and therapist should begin working on a plan to get off the meds as soon as possible. Having said that, there are some people who may need to be on medications for a very long time. For those types of people, they should be looking to be on the lowest dose required to effectively mitigate symptoms. Generally speaking, this is the best practice, when it comes to medication management. Make sure that, if you are someone who needs medication for your symptom severity, whomever is managing your prescriptions has this outlook. The reason for this is that medications can have side-effects that may be harmful and potentially hard to detect. Never be afraid to ask questions about medications and be aware of what you are putting into your body.

Finally, I would like to congratulate you for making it all the way through this book! Great job! I hope that this book has given you a deeper understanding of our complex relationship with anxiety. If you suffer from chronic, high levels of anxiety that make it hard to live a normal life, perhaps you now have some insight into what the causes might be. Hopefully, I have convinced you that, contrary to what Frank Herbert may have to say about anxiety, perhaps it isn't the "mind killer" that it's been made out to be. We just need to have a healthy relationship with it. I also hope that you will utilize the tools that I have given you in this book to manage your anxiety when you are feeling overwhelmed. I wish you the absolute best of luck on your journey through life. Feel free to join the Facebook group associated with this book, as there will be substantially more material posted there in the weeks and months to come, and feel free to subscribe to the YouTube channel as well. Goodbye and good luck!

Chapter Thirteen

References

American Psychiatric Association. (2022). *Diagnostic and statistical manual of mental disorders* (5th ed., text rev).

American Psychological Association. (2022). *Stress in America: Financial stress and the impact on mental health*. American Psychological Association.

Bandelow, B., & Michaelis, S. (2015). Epidemiology of anxiety disorders in the 21st century. *Dialogues in Clinical Neuroscience, 17*(3), 327–335.

Bail, C. A., Argyle, L., Chen, E. E., Brown, V., Bumpus, J. P., Hou, J., & Smith, S. (2018). Exposure to opposing views on social media can increase political polarization. *Proceedings of the National Academy of Sciences, 115*(37), 9216–9221.

Beck, A. T. (1976). *Cognitive therapy and the emotional disorders*. International Universities Press.

Bratman, G. N., Anderson, C. B., Berman, M. G., et al. (2015). Nature and mental health: An ecosystem service perspective. *Nature Communications, 6*, 6690.

Brooks, S. K., Webster, R. K., Wessely, S., Greenberg, N., & Rubin, G. J. (2020). The psychological impact of quarantine and how to reduce it: Rapid review of the evidence. *The Lancet, 395*(10227), 912–920.

Cacioppo, J. T., & Cacioppo, S. (2014). Social relationships and health: The toxic effects of perceived social isolation. *Social and Personality Psychology Compass, 8*(2), 58–72.

Carroll, K. M. (1998). Behavioral therapies for drug abuse. *The American Journal of Psychiatry, 155*(1), 27–37.

Centers for Disease Control and Prevention. (2021). *Fertility rates in the United States, 2021.*

Childs, E., & de Wit, H. (2017). The effects of cannabis on stress and anxiety: A review. *Psychopharmacology, 234*(9), 1333–1349.

Cox, W. M., & Klinger, E. (1988). A motivational model of alcohol use. *Journal of Abnormal Psychology, 97*(2), 168–180.

Davidson, R. J., Stafford, B., & Tompson, D. (2009). Mindfulness and craving: From the laboratory to the clinic. *Contemporary Clinical Trials, 30*(4), 341–346.

Engel, G. L. (1977). The need for a new medical model: A challenge for biomedicine. *Science, 196*(4286), 129–136.

Garfin, D. R., Silver, R. C., & Holman, E. A. (2020). The novel coronavirus (COVID-2019) outbreak: Amplification of public health consequences by media exposure. *Health Psychology, 39*(5), 355–357.

Garland, E. L., Hanley, A. W., Nakamura, Y., Barrett, J. W., Baker, A. K., Reese, S. E., Riquino, M. R., Froeliger, B., & Donaldson, G. W. (2022). Mindfulness-oriented recovery enhancement for co-occurring opioid misuse and chronic pain in primary care: A randomized clinical trial. *JAMA Internal Medicine.*

Goodwin, R. D., Weinberger, A. H., Kim, J. H., Wu, M., & Galea, S. (2020). Trends in anxiety among adults in the United States, 2008–2018: Rapid increases among young adults. *Journal of Psychiatric Research, 130,* 441–446.

Goyal, M., Singh, S., Sibinga, E., et al. (2014). Meditation programs for psychological stress and well-being: A systematic review and meta-analysis. *JAMA Internal Medicine, 174*(3), 357–368.

Hamer, M., & Chida, Y. (2008). Walking and primary prevention: a meta-analysis of prospective cohort studies. *British Journal of Sports Medicine, 42*(4), 238-243.

Herbert, F. (1965). *Dune.* Chilton Books.

Hirshkowitz, M., Whiton, K., Albert, S. M., et al. (2015). National Sleep Foundation's sleep time duration recommendations: Methodology and results summary. *Sleep Health, 1*(1), 40–43.

Holman, E. A., Garfin, D. R., & Silver, R. C. (2014). Media's role in broadcasting acute stress following the Boston Marathon bombings. *Proceedings of the National Academy of Sciences, 111*(1), 93–98.

Kabat-Zinn, J. (1990). *Full catastrophe living: Using the wisdom of your body and mind to face stress, pain, and illness*. Delacorte Press.

Kelly, J. F., Bergman, B., Hoeppner, B. B., Vilsaint, C., & White, W. L. (2017). Prevalence and pathways of recovery from drug and alcohol problems in the United States population: Implications for practice, research, and policy. *Drug and Alcohol Dependence, 181*, 162–169.

Kezelman, C. A., & Stavropoulos, P. (2012). The impact of trauma on emotional regulation and its therapeutic implications. *Australian & New Zealand Journal of Family Therapy, 33*(1), 7–20.

Lin, L. Y., Sidani, J. E., Shensa, A., Radovic, A., & Miller, E. (2016). Association Between Social Media Use and Depression Among U.S. Young Adults. *Depression and Anxiety, 33*(4), 323–331.

Meshi, D., Tamir, D. I., & Heekeren, H. R. (2015). The emerging neuroscience of social media. *Trends in Cognitive Sciences, 19*(12), 771–782.

Miller, W. R., & Rollnick, S. (2002). *Motivational interviewing: Preparing people for change* (2nd ed.). The Guilford Press.

National Center for Education Statistics. (2023). *Tuition costs of colleges and universities in the United States*.

O'Neil, A., Quirk, S., Housden, S., et al. (2014). Comparative efficacy of dietary patterns for mental health: A systematic review and meta-analysis. *Australian & New Zealand Journal of Psychiatry, 48*(10), 1083–1093.

Ouimette, P., Finney, J. W., & Moos, R. H. (1998). Twelve-step and mainstream addiction treatment: The role of client-treatment matching. *Journal of Substance Abuse Treatment, 15*(2), 121–130.

Pacula, R. L., Kilmer, B., & Wagenaar, A. C. (2014). Broadening access to marijuana and its impact on psychopathology and medical use. *Psychology of Addiction*, 110(2), 377–386.

Pennebaker, J. W., & Chung, C. K. (2007). Expressive Writing, Emotional Upheavals, and Health. In H. S. Friedman & R. C. Silver (Eds.), *Foundations of health psychology* (pp. 263–284). Oxford University Press.

Petruzzello, S. J., Landers, D. M., Hatfield, B. D., Kubitz, K. A., & Salazar, W. (1991). A meta-analysis on the anxiety-reducing effects of acute and chronic exercise. *Sports Medicine*, 11(3), 143-182.

Pew Research Center. (2021). *More than half of Americans say they have fewer than three close friends.*

Piercy, K. L., et al. (2018). The Physical Activity Guidelines for Americans. *JAMA, 320*(19), 2020–2028.

Pinker, S. (2018). *Enlightenment now: The case for reason, science, humanism, and progress.* Viking.

Przybylski, A. K., Murayama, K., DeHaan, C. R., & Gladwell, V. (2013). Motivational, emotional, and behavioral correlates of fear of missing out. *Computers in Human Behavior, 29*(4), 1841–1848.

Smyth, J. M., Stone, A. A., Hurewitz, A., & Kaell, A. (1999). Effects of writing about stressful experiences on symptom reduction in patients with asthma or rheumatoid arthritis: A randomized trial. *JAMA, 281*(14), 1304–1309.

Stuckey, H. L., & Nobel, J. (2010). The connection between art, healing, and public health: A review of current literature. *American Journal of Public Health, 100*(2), 254–263.

Tuithof, M., ten Have, M., Beekman, A., van Dorsselaer, S., Kleinjan, M., Schaufeli, W., & de Graaf, R. (2017). The interplay between emotional exhaustion, common mental disorders, functioning, and health care use in the working population. *Journal of Psychosomatic Research, 100*, 8–14.

Umberson, D., & Montez, J. K. (2010). Social relationships and health: A flashpoint for health policy. *Journal of Health and Social Behavior, 51*(Suppl), S54–S66.

U.S. Census Bureau. (2020). *Marriage and divorce rates in the United States.*

U.S. Census Bureau. (2023). *Median and average sales prices of new homes sold in the United States.*

Van Scoy, L. J., Snyder, B., Miller, E. L., Toyobo, O., Grewel, A., Ha, G., ... Lennon, R. P. (2021). Public anxiety and distrust due to perceived politicization and media sensationalism during early COVID-19 media messaging. *Journal of Communication in Healthcare, 14*(3), 193–205.

Ventriglio, A., Ricci, F., Torales, J., Castaldelli-Maia, J. M., Bener, A., Smith, A., & Liebrenz, M. (2024). Navigating a world in conflict: The mental health implications of contemporary geopolitical crises. *Industrial Psychiatry Journal, 33*(1), S268–S271.

Vogel, E. A., Rose, J. P., Roberts, L. R., & Eckles, K. (2014). Social comparison, social media, and self-esteem. *Psychology of Popular Media Culture, 3*(4), 206–222.

Volkow, N. D., Koob, G. F., & McLellan, A. T. (2009). Neurobiologic advances from the brain disease model of addiction. *The New England Journal of Medicine, 376*(4), 363–375.

Voshaar, R. C., Wessel, I., van den Hout, M. A., & Zitman, F. G. (2006). Patterns of benzodiazepine use in patients with anxiety disorders. *The British Journal of Psychiatry, 188*(6), 576–582.

Wipfli, B., Rethorst, C., & Landers, D. (2008). The anxiolytic effects of exercise: a meta-analysis of randomized trials and dose-response analysis. *Journal of Sport and Exercise Psychology*, 30(4), 392-410.

Zhao, G., Su, R., Miao, M., & Zhang, Y. (2018). The effects of daylight exposure on mood and circadian regulation: A systematic review. *Scientific Reports*, 8, 13986.

Made in the USA
Coppell, TX
21 January 2026

68974392R00098